PAEDIATRIC PSYCHOLOGY

Psychosocial Aspects of Diabetes

Children, adolescents and their families

Edited by

DEBORAH CHRISTIE

Consultant Clinical Psychologist
Honorary Reader in Paediatric and Adolescent Psychology
University College London Hospital NHS Foundation Trust

and

CLARISSA MARTIN

Consultant Paediatric Clinical Psychologist
Honorary Research Fellow, Loughborough University (LUCRED)
Staffordshire General Hospital

Series Editors
Angela Southall and Clarissa Martin

Foreword by
Francine R Kaufman MD
Distinguished Professor Emerita of Pediatrics and Communication
University of Southern California
Children's Hospital, Los Angeles

Radcliffe Publishing
London • New York

Radcliffe Publishing Ltd
33–41 Dallington Street
London
EC1V 0BB
United Kingdom

www.radcliffepublishing.com

———————————————————————

British Library Cataloguing in Publication Data

A catalogue record for this book is available from the British Library.

ISBN-13: 978 184619 513 6

Typeset by Darkriver Design, Auckland, New Zealand
Printed and bound by Cadmus Communications, USA

Contents

Series introduction

Whenever a child receives a diagnosis of a medical condition, numerous considerations are immediately brought to the fore, many of which are unique to children, including, of course, developmental, family and parenting issues. A child's cognitive, emotional, behavioural and social functioning may be significantly affected by their illness. Most significantly, just as the child is affected by their illness, so is the course of the illness affected by the child. This simple understanding and the success of paediatric psychologists in communicating and demonstrating it has led to the growth of paediatric psychology in children's wards, outpatient departments, community clinics and health centres around the world. Indeed, it is the propensity of the paediatric psychology team to make a difference to the child and their treatment that has led to widespread acknowledgement of the value that paediatric psychology brings.

Paediatric psychology is essentially the application of psychological theory, research and practice to children with medical conditions and health-related concerns. It takes a 'whole child' approach and is developmentally focused. Practice is most often multidisciplinary and focuses on the understanding of physical, psychosocial and neuropsychological aspects of health and illness, and how these impact on each other. The scope of paediatric psychology is extensive and encompasses many treatment areas ranging from adjustment to illness, coping with invasive medical procedures and pain management to adherence to treatment, children with chronic conditions and palliative care, to name just a few, as well as the prevention of illness among healthy children (Roberts et al., 1984).

As a specialty, paediatric psychology has a surprisingly long history. Soon after the emergence of psychology as a discipline in the nineteenth century, it was suggested that psychologists and paediatricians would benefit from mutual collaboration (Witmer, 1907). These psychologists worked alongside paediatricians and shared with them a developmental perspective; they came to be described as 'paediatric psychologists' (Wright, 1967). These early paediatric psychologists helped establish that children with health and developmental problems had significant needs, which, though similar to one another, were different to those with psychiatric diagnoses. In the United States, the Society of Pediatric Psychology was founded to meet those needs (Wright, 1967). In the United Kingdom, paediatric psychology developed out of the discipline of clinical psychology and continues to be located within the category of *clinical child psychologists working in medical healthcare settings*, under the auspices of the British Psychological Society.

Recent policy emphases in the United Kingdom have highlighted the needs of children and young people with long-term conditions and the importance of providing them with good mental health input to maximise emotional well-being and minimise problems.[1] These policies emphasise that such support should be an integral part of the service a child receives in hospital and high-light the imperative on hospitals to ensure staff have an understanding of how to assess the emotional well-being of children and address any needs that are identified.[2] Elsewhere in Europe, mental health has also come to be empha-sised as an essential ingredient in health and well-being, not just for children but for everyone. This is perhaps best exemplified by the European Union's slogan, 'There is no health without mental health' (Lavikainen *et al.*, 2000).

The Paediatric Psychology series to which this book belongs was conceived as a way of sharing with readers salient ideas from applied research and practice that would be experienced as helpful to others in their own practice. A series of books was planned, each focusing on a different topic within paediatric psy-chology, with the overall aim of raising awareness among health professionals of the concomitant psychological and psychosocial aspects of child ill health and chronic illness.

The series has a deliberately international focus, which reflects the paedi-atric psychology community and brings together material that is otherwise unavailable in this form. The accompanying electronic toolkit offers practical, usable support to practitioners, as well as an opportunity to contribute to the developing knowledge base. It is our hope that the books will prove to be an inspiring and reliable resource for day-to-day paediatric practice.

Angela Southall
Clarissa Martin

---

1 Department of Health (2004) *National Service Framework (NSF) for children young people and maternity services: children and young people who are ill. Standard 6.* London: DoH.
2 Department of Health (2003) *National Service Framework (NSF) for children at hospital. Standard 7.* London: DoH.

REFERENCES

Lavikainen J, Lahtinen E, Lehtinen V, editors. *Public Health Approach on Mental Health in Europe.* National Research and Development Centre for Welfare and Health, STAKES Ministry of Social Affairs and Health; 2000.

Roberts MC, Maddux JE, Wright L. Developmental perspectives in behavioral health. In: Matarazzo JD, Miller NE, Weiss SM, *et al.*, editors. *Behavioral Health: a handbook of health enhancement and disease prevention.* New York, NY: Wiley; 1984.

Wright L. The pediatric psychologist: a role model. *Am Psychol.* 1967; **22**(4): 323–5.

Witmer L. Clinical psychology. *Psychol Clinic.* 1907; **1**(1): 1–9.

Dedicated to Dr J Houghton PhD

This series is dedicated to Dr Judith Houghton PhD,
Consultant Clinical Psychologist and first elected chair
(2001–06) of the British Psychological Society – Paediatric
Psychology National Committee (BPS-PPNC) in gratitude
and acknowledgement for her outstanding contribution
to the development of Paediatric Psychology in the UK.

Foreword

Diabetes has a unique impact on children and their families. The daily life of children and youth is affected by the rigours of the diabetes regimen and the need to frequently monitor glucose levels, give glucose-lowering agents and balance the effect of activity and food. Despite this, paediatric patients must still strive to reach the normal developmental milestones of childhood and adolescence, succeed in school and develop eventual autonomy. To accomplish these tasks, an organised system of diabetes care utilising a multidisciplinary team versed in paediatric and psychological issues must be in place to assure optimal physical and emotional health for the affected child.

The treatment of type 1 diabetes in children and youth has become increasingly complex over the last few decades. There are increasing numbers of insulin preparations, including rapid- and long-acting or basal analogues, multiple methodologies to monitor glucose levels either on an intermittent or continuous basis, conventional and intensive ways to deliver insulin and well-defined goals and outcome measures. For the most part, healthcare providers determine which therapies they will prescribe for their patients at diagnosis, and at what pace they may change or advance therapies as time goes on. However, as patients and their families gain knowledge, skills and experience, they hopefully contribute more to therapeutic decision-making and develop a true partnership with their providers, so that their individual capabilities and aspirations can play a role in how they manage diabetes in the context of their family, their child's developmental stage and within the framework of their mental health and emotional well-being. Key to success for the therapeutic alliance between providers and patients/families is awareness that diabetes management can only be successful if psychosocial needs are assessed and addressed.

The purpose of this edition, *Psychosocial Aspects of Diabetes: children, adolescent and their families*, edited by Deborah Christie and Clarissa Martin, from the series on Paediatric Psychology, is to inform the reader about how diabetes affects children/families, how children's/families' characteristics influence diabetes, the role of the multidisciplinary team and of diabetes education, and what psychological approaches and tools are available to use with patients. The well-known authors who have contributed to this compendium are leaders in the field of paediatric diabetes. Collectively, they offer a comprehensive, well-written review, and information that will enable the reader to develop new ways to approach their patients/families. This series offers the hope that together we can all make the journey with diabetes more tolerable and successful for children, youth and their families, who we all care for today and who we will care for in the future. As knowledge about diabetes and its treatment options expand, we must not forget that the most important thing we must guarantee our patients is that we will do everything we can to enable them to accept and adjust to having a chronic, demanding illness and to reach adulthood with as little adverse impact on their psychological and physical well-being as possible.

Francine Ratner Kaufman MD
Distinguished Professor Emerita of Pediatrics and
Communications, University of Southern California
The Center for Diabetes, Endocrinology & Metabolism,
Children's Hospital, Los Angeles
Chief Medical Officer and VP of Global Clinical, Medical
and Health Affairs, Medtronic Diabetes
January 2012

About the editors

Deborah Christie is a Consultant Clinical Psychologist and Honorary Reader in Paediatric and Adolescent Psychology. She is the clinical lead for paediatric and adolescent psychology at the University College London Hospital's NHS Foundation Trust. She is an international presenter and trainer in motivational and solution-focused therapies. She works with multidisciplinary teams to help them engage and communicate effectively with children, young people and families who are searching for ways to live with chronic illness including diabetes, obesity, arthritis, chronic fatigue and chronic pain syndromes. Research interests include evaluating effective multidisciplinary interventions for diabetes and obesity in children and adolescents, the development of quality of life measures in chronic illness and outcomes of meningitis in children and adolescent survivors. Awards include the Association for the Study of Obesity Best Practice Award (2001), the Society for Adolescent Medicine Diabetes Award in Adolescent Health (2001) and the award for Outstanding Scientific Achievement in Clinical Health Psychology (2004). She has published over 90 peer-reviewed papers and chapters.

Clarissa Martin is Consultant Clinical Psychologist in Paediatrics and Honorary Research Fellow at the Centre for Research in Eating Disorders at Loughborough University (LUCRED) in the United Kingdom, where she is the clinical lead for the feeding centre. She is a specialist in children's feeding disorders and has pioneered multidisciplinary intensive intervention for children with severe feeding disorders in a general hospital setting. She also leads a CAMHS Paediatric Psychology specialty and is involved in multidisciplinary clinics (diabetes and gastroenterology) helping children, young people and their families to adapt to the illness. She is also active in collaborative, interdisciplinary work in both community and acute settings. She has extensive experience of developing and delivering training to health professionals to support the enhancement of their skills in psychosocial aspects of paediatric care. She is known for her national and international conference contributions and is the author of a number of peer-reviewed papers in the area of diabetes and gastroenterology. She is co-editor, with Angela Southall, of this series in Paediatric Psychology, the first of its kind in the UK.

List of contributors

Christina Akré
Anthropologist and researcher in
  adolescent health
University Institute of Social and
  Preventive Medicine
Centre Hospitalier Universitaire Vaudois
Lausanne, Switzerland

Katherine Barnard
Health Psychologist, NETSCC
University of Southampton
Southampton, UK

Sue Channon
Consultant Clinical Psychologist
Children's Centre, St David's Hospital
Cardiff
Wales

Dr Deborah Christie
Consultant Clinical Psychologist
Honorary Reader in Paediatric and
  Adolescent Psychology
University College London Hospital
  NHS Foundation Trust
London, UK

Susie Colville
Research Assistant
Child and Adolescent Psychological
  Services
University College London Hospital
  NHS Foundation Trust
London, UK

Amber Daigre
Postdoctoral Scholar in Pediatric
  Psychology
University of Miami
Mailman Center for Child Development
Miami, FL

Dr Carine De Beaufort
Consultant in Paediatric Endocrinology
Clinique de Pediatrique de Luxembourg
Luxembourg

Prof Alan Delamater
Professor of Pediatrics & Psychology
Director of Clinical Psychology
University of Miami Miller School of
  Medicine
Mailman Centre for Child Development
Dept of Pediatrics – Division of Clinical
  Psychology
Miami, FL

Glenda Fredman
Consultant Clinical Psychologist
University College London Hospital
  NHS Foundation Trust
London, UK

Rebecca Gebert
Credentialed Diabetes Educator
Royal Children's Hospital
Victoria, Australia

Dr Helena Gleeson
Hon Consultant in Adolescent
  Endocrinology
Royal Manchester Children's Hospital
Manchester, UK

Dr Angela Griffin
Montrose
Lyndhurst
Hants

Dr Ragnar Hanas
Consultant Paediatrician
Department of Paediatrics
Uddevalla Hospital
Uddevalla
Sweden

Clarissa Martin
Consultant Paediatric Clinical
  Psychologist
Honorary Research Fellow.
  Loughborough University
Paediatric Psychology Specialty
Staffordshire General Hospital
Stafford
UK

Dr Janet McDonagh
Consultant Rheumatologist
Clinical Senior Lecturer in Paediatric and
  Adolescent Rheumatology
Institute of Child Health
Birmingham Children's Hospital NHS
  Foundation Trust
Birmingham, UK

Julia Núñez
Licenciada en Psycologia
Universidad de Valencia
Valencia
Spain

Prof Anna Maria Patino-Fernandez
Assistant Professor of Clinical Pediatrics
University of Miami Miller School of
  Medicine
Mailman Centre for Child Development
Dept of Pediatrics – Division of Clinical
  Psychology
Miami, FL

Elizabeth Pulgaron
Assistant Professor of Clinical Pediatrics
University of Miami Miller School of
  Medicine
Miami, FL

Katie Ridge
Department of Psychological Medicine
Institute of Psychiatry
London, UK

Daniel Royo
Licenciado en Psychologia
Asociación Valenciana Diabetes
Valencia
Spain

Joan-Carles Surís
Chef d'unité
Groupe de recherche sur la santé des
  adolescents (GRSA)
Institut universitaire de médecine sociale
  et préventive (IUMSP)
Epalinges
Switzerland

Rebecca Thompson
Diabetes Clinical Nurse Specialist
University College London Hospital
  NHS Foundation Trust
London, UK

Prof Janet Treasure
Dept Academic Psychiatry, Bermondsey
  Wing
Guy's Hospital
London, UK

Russell Viner
Reader in Adolescent Medicine and
  Consultant in Endocrinology
Institute of Child Health
General Paediatric and Adolescent Unit
London, UK

Introduction

Including a book on the psychosocial aspects of paediatric diabetes as part of the Paediatric Psychology series seemed essential. Diabetes is a metabolic condition recognised since ancient times (Patlak, 2002) and is now one of the leading chronic diseases of childhood in the world.

The observation of diabetes-related symptoms such as the sweetness of urine and frequency of passing urine have been found in ancient texts from Egyptian, Chinese, Greek and Persian cultures. However, it was not until the middle of the nineteenth century when the relationship between the pancreas and diabetes was highlighted by scientific research. The revolutionary work of Banting and Macleod resulting in the availability of treatment with insulin in 1922 earned them a Nobel Prize for their discovery. Since then research has expanded our knowledge of diabetes, its complications, revolutionised its management through the advances in insulin therapy and the techniques for its administration, and has enabled the translation of research findings into practical and clinical action (Stetson, Ruggiero and Jack, 2010). At the beginning of the century the World Health Organization (WHO) reported at least 171 million people worldwide suffered from diabetes (Wild et al., 2004). This figure increased to 285 million in 2010 which was 40 million more than the International Diabetes Federation's (IDF) estimate in 2007. By 2030, it is expected that this number will almost double with an estimated 366 million children, adolescents and adults diagnosed with diabetes, approximately 4.4% of the population (Wild et al., 2004). The IDF (2009) have estimated a 3% worldwide annual increase in diabetes which would put the European region in second place in worldwide ranking.

Two international collaborative projects sponsored by WHO, the EURODIAB (Patterson et al., 2009) and the Diabetes Mondiale study (DIAMOND, 2006) addressed the need for more standardised data to be collected. Both included population data from multisite centres and from several countries. The DIAMOND study included 75.1 million people under 14 years of age diagnosed with diabetes between 1990-94 (Lipton, 2007). More recently, Karvonen and colleagues (2000) have investigated the patterns of worldwide incidence of type 1 diabetes in children. They found a huge between-population variation and concluded that the incidence was even greater than previously described. All the figures emphasise the epidemic nature of diabetes (Unwin, Gan and Whiting, 2010).

International efforts have also been made to improve the care of people suffering from diabetes in terms of life expectancy, quality of life and the provision of health systems and services. These efforts were reflected in the St Vincent Declaration (1989) where representatives of the WHO, IDF, European Health Departments and patients from several countries met and agreed a set of minimum standards for diabetes care. This document's unanimous agreement has encouraged European countries to develop national policies and programmes to improve treatment and care for people living with diabetes (Piwernetz et al., 1993). This initiative was further supported by the United Nations Organization resolution 61/225 in 2006 which encouraged countries to develop national policies that included psychosocial aspects of paediatric diabetes care.

In the UK in 1994 the Division of Clinical Psychology (DCP) of the British Psychological Society (BPS) published a briefing paper about clinical psychology services, describing the psychological challenges of living with diabetes and how psychologists can work to facilitate adjustment to these challenges. It also addressed their role in providing consultancy for diabetes medical teams with recommendations for service specifications. The UK Department of Health identified the need for improved access to specialist services to support the physical, psychological, educational and social needs of the 20 000 children and young people under 15 with diabetes in the UK (Datta, 2003; *Making Every Young Person with Diabetes Matter*, DoH, 2007; *Emotional and Psychological Support and Care in Diabetes*, NHS Diabetes/Diabetes UK, 2010). Current UK guidelines for the diagnosis and management of type 1 diabetes in children, young people and adults, published by the National Institute for Health and Clinical Excellence (NICE, 2010), are clear that children and young people with diabetes are at risk of suffering greater psychological problems than other children and are in need of psychosocial support. Access to services to help them with these issues should be offered by all diabetes teams.

It is within this context that this book was created to offer health professionals, students and the public up-to-date research and clinical practice in the psychological and social aspects of paediatric and adolescent diabetes. The book has been written in three parts: Part I focuses on understanding the emotional and behavioural impact of diabetes on children, young people and their families; Part II describes empirical and evidence-based clinical approaches for management and intervention; and Part III includes tools, tips and techniques for clinical practice and service development.

Hanas in Chapter 1 provides a macro systems perspective offering a global understanding of diabetes and its worldwide prevalence and incidence. Martin, Núñez and Royo in Chapter 2 describe the emotional and social impact that a diagnosis of diabetes creates for children, young people, their families and the wider family system. In Chapter 3, De Beaufort and Barnard review the prevalence and incidence of the most common forms of emotional distress experienced by children and young people. The chapter focuses on how to recognise anxiety and depression as well as thinking about the emotional impact on parents and how this can influence their ability to manage diabetes safely. Delamater, Patino-Fernandez, Pulgaron and Daigre in Chapter 4 address the challenges created by the complex demands of the diabetes regimen. The chapter describes the different perspectives of the children, young people, families and healthcare professionals and the issues that affect optimal adherence to the regimen. The impact of hypoglycaemia and hyperglycaemia on neuropsychological functioning and school performance that results from less than optimal control is extensively reviewed by Griffin and Christie in Chapter 5. Surís and Akré in Chapter 6 describe normal exploratory behaviours in adolescence and review the extent to which diabetes has an impact on these risk behaviours.

In Part II the authors address the clinical management of diabetes and the particular challenges that exist when working with children and adolescents. In Chapter 7, Thompson, Delamater, Gebert and Christie review the different roles played by different healthcare professionals and summarise the international evidence-based consensus for the need for coordinated multidisciplinary provision of diabetes care. Viner in Chapter 8 discusses the different treatment regimes that teams use and the metabolic, psychological and social implications these can have for the child, young person and their family. A comprehensive review of the current guidelines and international evidence for structured education is provided by Thompson in Chapter 9, followed by Gebert's review in Chapter 10 of the specific and unique contribution the diabetes educator can make.

Psychological approaches that have been shown experimentally and empirically to be helpful for children, young people and families who get tripped up by diabetes are discussed in Chapters 11 and 12. The importance of motivational interviewing is referred to in Chapter 11. Channon looks at how ambivalence in relation to diabetes self-care can create difficulties for children and young people as well as healthcare professionals. Channon discusses the background and theory to motivational interviewing as well as providing case vignettes and examples of how to use motivational approaches to invite people to consider change, as well as to put it into practice. Christie also highlights the importance of engagement and motivation as a key component in behaviour change and in Chapter 12 provides an example of solution-focused therapy, as well as clinical descriptions of how non-psychologists in the healthcare team can use brief therapy approaches to work alongside families in a collaborative and engaging manner.

The difficulty of managing co-morbidities is highlighted in Chapter 13 where Treasure and Ridge review the assessment and management of diabetes and eating disorders in adolescents. Once again vignettes highlight clinical dilemmas and treatment approaches. Finally, in Chapter 14 Gleeson and McDonagh discuss the literature on the urgent need for appropriate and carefully thought out transitional care for young people with diabetes. The authors discuss how failure to ensure adequate transitional support as young people move to adult services can compromise their engagement in the healthcare service and, ultimately, impact upon long-term health and well-being.

In Part III a compendium of tools, tips and techniques that can be used to help service development and clinical practice is presented. Colville provides an extensive list of diagnostic tools that can be used for assessment of behaviour, depression, anxiety and Quality of Life in children and young people with diabetes. Delamater, Patino-Fernandez, Pulgaron and Daigre have also compiled specific measures of regimen adherence. Griffin offers assessment approaches and intervention strategies for children and young people who are struggling at school and who may have cognitive difficulties connected with poor metabolic control. Finally, Gleeson and McDonagh provide a toolkit for developing transition services.

As healthcare professionals we are always inspired by the hope, determination and resilience that we come across working with children, young people and their parents who live every day of their lives with the challenges and opportunities that diabetes can bring. We and our fellow authors couldn't have written this book without the inspiration that these families give us in our professional lives, and hope that it will inspire you to find new ideas and suggestions to help you in your work with the children, young people and families that you work with.

Deborah Christie and Clarissa Martin
January 2012

REFERENCES

British Psychological Society (BPS), Division of Clinical Psychology (DCP). *Purchasing Clinical Psychology Services for People with Diabetes Mellitus*. Briefing Paper Number 4. Leicester: British Psychological Society; 1994.

Datta J. *Moving Up With Diabetes*. London: National Children's Bureau; 2003.

Department of Health. *Making Every Young Person with Diabetes Matter*. London: Department of Health; 2007. Available at: www.dh.gov.uk/en/Publicationsandstatistics/Publications/PublicationsPolicyAndGuidance/DH_073674 (accessed 21 January 2012).

DIAMOND Project Group. Incidence and trends of childhood type 1 diabetes worldwide, 1990–1999. *Diabet Med*. 2006; **23**(8): 857–66.

International Diabetes Federation (IDF). Diabetes, facts and figures. *Diabetes Atlas*. 4th ed. Brussels: International Diabetes Federation; 2009. Available at: www.diabetesatlas.org

International Diabetes Federation (IDF). *The Diabetes Atlas*. 3rd ed. Brussels: International Diabetes Federation; 2006.

Karvonen M, Viit-Kajander M, Moltchanova E, *et al*. Incidence of childhood type 1 diabetes worldwide. *Diabetes Care*. 2000; **23**(10): 1516–26.

Lipton RB. Incidence of diabetes in children and youth: tracking a moving target. *JAMA*. 2007; **297**(24): 2760–2.

NHS Diabetes/Diabetes UK. *Emotional and Psychological Support and Care in Diabetes*. Report from the Emotional and Psychological Support Working Group. 2010. Available at: www.diabetes.nhs.uk/areas_of_care/emotional_and_psychological_support/ (accessed 23 January 2012).

NICE website: www.nice.org.uk/CG015NICEguideline; 2010.

Patlak M. New weapons to combat an ancient disease: treating diabetes. *FASEB J*. 2002; **16**(14): 1853.

Patterson C, Dahlquist G, Gyürüs E, *et al*. EURODIAB Study Group. Incidence trends for childhood type 1 diabetes in Europe during 1989–2003 and predicted new cases 2005–20: a multicentre prospective registration study. *Lancet*. 2009; **373**: 2027–33.

Piwernetz K, Home P, Snorgaard O, *et al*. Monitoring the targets of the St Vincent Declaration and the implementation of quality management in diabetes care: the DIABCARE initiative. The DIABCARE Monitoring Group of the St Vincent Declaration Steering Committee. *Diabet Med*. 1993; **10**(4): 371–7.

Stetson B, Ruggiero L, Jack L. Strategies for improving the acquisition and integration of evidence into diabetes care. *Diabetes Spectrum*. 2010; **23**(4): 246–53.

Unwin N, Gan D, Whiting D. The IDF Diabetes Atlas: providing evidence, raising awareness and promoting action. *Diabet Res Clin Pract*. 2010; **87**: 2–3.

Wild S, Roglic G, Green A, *et al*. Global prevalence of diabetes: estimates for 2000 and projections for 2030. *Diabetes Care*. 2004; **27**(5): 1047–53.

PART I

Understanding Diabetes

CHAPTER 1

A global perspective on childhood diabetes: worldwide prevalence and incidence

Ragnar Hanas

INTRODUCTION

Diabetes mellitus is a group of metabolic conditions characterised by chronic hyperglycaemia (high blood glucose) resulting from defaults in insulin secretion, insulin action or both. Insulin allows glucose in the bloodstream to enter into cells in order to be converted into energy. When there is insufficient insulin, the cells start to produce ketones, ultimately causing ketoacidosis. This can cause coma and, ultimately, death. The abnormalities in carbohydrate, fat and protein metabolism found in diabetes are due to inadequate action of insulin on target organs (Craig *et al.*, 2009). Diagnostic criteria for diabetes are based on blood glucose levels and the presence or absence of symptoms (*see* Table 1.1).

Prevalence and incidence figures vary across countries. For example, in the United Kingdom there are at least 20 000 children under 15 years of age with diabetes of all types (Jefferson *et al.*, 2003). In the United States, approximately 13 000 new cases of diabetes are diagnosed in children every year (Klingensmith *et al.*, 2003). Some 154 000 US citizens under the age of 19 years have diabetes (one out of every 523 young persons), making this the second most common chronic disease in school-age children – the first being asthma (Liese *et al.*, 2006).

This chapter introduces diabetes and the different types from a global perspective. World prevalence and incidence figures for diabetes are presented and discussed, as well as the different resources that countries may employ in its management.

TABLE 1.1 Criteria for the diagnosis of diabetes mellitus (ADA, 2010; WHO, 1999; reproduced from Craig *et al.*, 2009)

1.	Symptoms of diabetes plus casual plasma glucose concentration ≥ 11.1 mmol/L (200 mg/dL).*
	Casual is defined as any time of day without regard to time since last meal.
	or
2.	Fasting plasma glucose ≥ 7.0 mmol/L (≥ 126 mg/dL).**
	Fasting is defined as no caloric intake for at least 8 h.
	or
3.	2-hr postload glucose ≥ 11.1 mmol/L (≥ 200 mg/dL) during an OGTT.
	The test should be performed as described by WHO (86), using a glucose load containing the equivalent of 75 g anhydrous glucose dissolved in water or 1.75 g/kg of body weight to a maximum of 75 g (65).

* Corresponding values (mmol/L) are ≥ 10.0 for venous whole blood and ≥ 11.1 for capillary whole blood and **≥ 6.3 for both venous and capillary whole blood.

DIFFERENT TYPES OF DIABETES
Type 1
Mankind has known diabetes mellitus, usually referred to simply as 'diabetes', since ancient times. Diabetes means 'flowing through' and mellitus means 'sweet as honey'. Egyptian hieroglyphic findings from 1550 BC illustrate the symptoms of diabetes. In the past, diabetes was diagnosed by tasting the urine of the patient. No effective treatment was available. Before insulin was discovered, type 1 diabetes always resulted in death, usually quite quickly.

In type 1 diabetes, an autoimmune process destroys the insulin-producing cells of the pancreas. When tested, most children with new-onset diabetes are positive for pancreatic autoantibodies. This eventually leads to a total loss of insulin production. Type 1 diabetes is insulin-dependent, meaning that treatment with insulin is necessary from the time the disease is first diagnosed. Insulin is given by injection, with syringes increasingly being replaced by insulin pens. Twice-daily injections have for a long time been the traditional method of treating diabetes. To provide a more physiological insulin profile, short-acting insulin needs to be given with each meal, and there is also a need for a long-acting insulin (basal insulin) to be given once or twice daily through multiple daily injections (MDIs). In many centres, it is routine to begin with MDIs at the time of diagnosis. Most school-age children learn quickly how to give themselves injections. The average age for learning how to self-inject is around 8 years old (Wysocki *et al.*, 1996). However, for some children and adolescents, injecting insulin remains unbearable even after many years of living with diabetes. In one paediatric study, 8.3% of subjects scored themselves as having a pronounced needle phobia (Hanas and Ludvigsson, 1997).

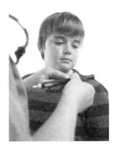

Boy being shown insulin injection device

Managing insulin delivery

There is a wide range of devices that have been developed to help improve the experience of injecting insulin. For example, indwelling catheters (Insuflon, I-port) may be used to help decrease injection pain for those who are new to injections, and they can be especially useful when multiple injections are used from the onset of diabetes (Hanas *et al.*, 2002). Insulin pens, often used for MDIs, deliver insulin more accurately (Lteif *et al.*, 1999) and are easier to handle than syringes (Graff and McClanahan, 1998), while injection aids (PenMate) for pens insert the needle automatically (Diglas *et al.*, 1998). Two pens have a memory, which can be used as a reminder that insulin has been injected (or forgotten): the HumaPen Memoir has 16 memories and the NovoPen Echo has one. Parents can check the memory and help their child or teenager find strategies to remember their doses. Forgetting only two doses of insulin per week has been found to raise glycated haemoglobin (HbA$_{1c}$)[1] by as much as 0.5% (Burdick *et al.*, 2004).

   An alternative to injections is the use of insulin pump therapy, also called continuous subcutaneous insulin infusion (CSII). This is increasing in use in developing countries. A small pump (about the size of a pager) delivers a continuous infusion of short-acting insulin via an indwelling subcutaneous catheter. With this type of therapy, no long-acting insulin is used, as the basal infusion rate can be adjusted to match the individual's varying needs during the day and night. The pump can deliver extra insulin (bolus) when eating or when

---

1   HbA$_{1c}$ is a form of haemoglobin measured to identify the concentration of glucose over periods of time. It is used as a marker for average blood glucose levels. Higher amounts of HbA$_{1c}$ are indicators of poorly controlled blood glucose levels.

TABLE 1.2 Different modes of insulin delivery

Frequency	Consists of	Type of delivery
Twice-daily injections	Mixture of regular short- or rapid-acting insulin and intermediate-acting basal insulin	Mixed in syringe or pre-mixed in an insulin pen
Three times daily injections	Morning injection of mixture of regular short- or rapid- and intermediate-acting insulins before breakfast; rapid-acting or regular short-acting insulin alone before afternoon snack or main evening meal; intermediate-acting insulin before bed	Mixed in syringe or pre-mixed in an insulin pen in morning Syringe or pen for the other injections
Multiple daily injections	Basal insulin once or twice daily and rapid- or regular short-acting insulin before each meal	Usually insulin pens, but syringes can also be used
Continuous subcutaneous insulin infusion	Only rapid-acting (or short-acting) insulin is used in the pump The basal rate used in the pump substitutes for injection of basal insulin Bolus doses of insulin are given before each meal Rapid- or regular short-acting insulin is used	Insulin pump, bolus doses are delivered by pressing the buttons on the pump

the blood glucose is high by pressing the pump buttons. Parents report that their children achieve CSII skill mastery at a mean age of 12.5 years (Weissberg-Benchell *et al.*, 2007). The use of insulin pumps in very young children has become established in many centres, and many now begin with insulin pumps from the onset of diabetes (Phillip *et al.*, 2007). All insulin pumps have extensive memory capabilities, and it is possible to download details of previous bolus doses and basal rates for more than a month. This is very helpful during consultations, and it creates opportunities for discussions about how a young

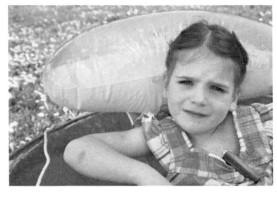

A little girl plays happily in the sunshine: her insulin
pump is visible at the neckline of her dress

person or parent is managing the diabetes regimen. Using insulin pumps from the onset of diabetes in the age group 7–17 years has been shown to give better scores on the Diabetes Treatment Satisfaction Scale (Bradley, 1994), but has not shown improvement in glycaemic control (Skogsberg *et al.*, 2008). Parents whose children are younger than 12 years of age have reported more freedom, flexibility and spontaneity in their lives, as well as reduced parental stress and worry regarding their child's overall care, when switching from MDIs to CSII (Sullivan-Bolyai *et al.*, 2004).

Managing diabetes in school

MDIs and pump therapy both require an insulin dose to be taken when the child has lunch at school. Whereas older children should be able to manage this by themselves, younger children need help, both with taking insulin and with measuring blood glucose. Children who have adequate support from their school are reported to have a better quality of life and to be less burdened by their condition (Peyrot and Aanstoot, 2008). In a Swedish survey (Särnblad *et al.*, 2009), 21% of the parents regularly gave less insulin than needed in the morning because of fear of hypoglycaemia during school time, and 40% of the children were not sure if they could get help from school personnel in the event of hypoglycaemia.

Type 2

In type 2 diabetes, the ability to produce insulin does not disappear completely, but the body becomes increasingly resistant to insulin. The medication used for treating type 2 diabetes acts by increasing the body's sensitivity to insulin, or by increasing the release of insulin from the pancreas. Diet, exercise and obesity management are also very important when treating type 2 diabetes. It is rare for insulin injections to be necessary in the early stages of type 2 diabetes, except when there is excessive hyperglycaemia or ketoacidosis at diagnosis. Although type 2 diabetes is also called non-insulin-dependent diabetes, many people need treatment with insulin at a later stage, in much the same way as people with type 1 diabetes.

An increasing number of reports from the United States, Japan, the United Kingdom and other parts of the industrialised world indicate that overweight teenagers are now beginning to develop type 2 diabetes. This appears to be more common in girls than in boys (Ehtisham *et al.*, 2000). In the United States, type 2 diabetes and heart disease among young and middle-aged people in members of the Native American population is reaching epidemic proportions (Rosenbloom, 2000). In certain groups, the number of cases of type 2 diabetes as a proportion of the total number of newly diagnosed diabetes among children and adolescents is extremely high. Type 2 diabetes is rare under the age of 9 years, but in older children the proportion of type 2 diabetes varies greatly among racial and ethnic groups (Native American, 76%; Asian/Pacific Islander, 40%; African American, 33%; Hispanic, 22%; non-Hispanic white, 6%; as reported by Liese *et al.* (2006)).

BOX 1.1 Risk factors for type 2 diabetes in children and young people (Ehtisham *et al.*, 2000; Rosenbloom, 2000)

- Low birth weight.
- Type 2 diabetes in the family.
- Ethnic origin.[2]
- A diet that is high in fat and low in fibre.
- Being overweight.
- Lack of exercise.
- High blood pressure.
- Acanthosis nigricans (a dark, velvety discoloration of the skin).

Monogenic diabetes

Monogenic diabetes results from the inheritance of a mutation or mutations in a single gene. It may be dominantly or recessively inherited or it may be a de novo mutation and hence a spontaneous case. In children, almost all monogenic diabetes results from mutations in genes that regulate beta-cell function in the pancreas, although diabetes can, rarely, occur from mutations, resulting in very severe insulin resistance (Hattersley *et al.*, 2009). Monogenic diabetes is associated with a strong family history of diabetes, and taking a genetic test should be considered if diabetes is present in several generations of a family. Genetic testing can now identify many clinically identified subgroups of diabetes. The different types of MODY (maturity-onset diabetes of the young) and neonatal diabetes have been classified into subcategories. One type of MODY (MODY2) has a modest increase in blood glucose levels, which often does not need any treatment at all besides a diet. People with MODY2 seldom get complications from their diabetes. Some forms of MODY can be treated successfully with antidiabetic drugs, while people with other forms of MODY are very likely to need insulin.

A special form of diabetes has been discovered in approximately half of the children with an onset of permanent diabetes under the age of 6 months

---

2   Canadian and US First Nations peoples, Hispanic, African American, Japanese, Pacific Islander, Asian and Middle Eastern.

(Slingerland *et al.*, 2009). The difficulty in secreting insulin is caused by a mutation responsible for regulating the release of insulin from the beta cells. This type of diabetes can be treated with a high dose of a class of the antidiabetic drug sulphonylurea (Hattersley and Ashcroft, 2005).

TABLE 1.3 Clinical characteristics of type 1 diabetes, type 2 diabetes and monogenic diabetes in children and adolescents (reproduced from Craig *et al.*, 2009)

Characteristic	Type 1	Type 2	Monogenic
Genetics	Polygenic	Polygenic	Monogenic
Age of onset	6 months to young adulthood	Usually pubertal (or later)	Often post-pubertal except glucokinase and neonatal diabetes
Clinical presentation	Most often acute, rapid	Variable; from slow, mild (often insidious) to severe	Variable (may be incidental in glucokinase)
Associations			
Autoimmunity	Yes	No	No
Ketosis	Common	Uncommon	Common in neonatal diabetes, rare in other forms
Obesity	Population frequency	Increased frequency	Population frequency
Acanthosis nigricans	No	Yes	No
Frequency (% of all diabetes in young people)	Usually 90%+	Most countries < 10% Japan (60%–80%)	1%–3%
Parent with diabetes	24%	80%	90%

Other forms of diabetes

Secondary diabetes can also result when the pancreas is affected directly or indirectly by other conditions (e.g. cancer or pancreatitis). Cystic fibrosis–related diabetes (CFRD) is the most common co-morbidity in cystic fibrosis. There are important differences between CFRD and both type 1 and type 2 diabetes; these differences necessitate a unique approach to diagnosis and management. Cystic fibrosis results in thick, viscous secretions causing obstructive damage to the pancreas with progressive fibrosis and fatty infiltration (O'Riordan *et al.*, 2009). In these cases, the dysfunction of the beta cells is not caused by autoimmunity.

PREVALENCE AND INCIDENCE IN DIFFERENT COUNTRIES

Time trends of incidence

Finland has the highest incidence of childhood diabetes in the world, at 64.2 per 100 000 per year in 2005 (Harjutsalo *et al.*, 2008), followed by Sardinia, Canada and Sweden. There are huge discrepancies in incidence among different parts of the world. For example, Peru has an incidence of 0.4 per 100 000 (Karvonen *et al.*, 2000), which is one-hundredth of that in Sweden. The incidence of type 1 diabetes with onset in childhood is rapidly increasing in many countries in the world. The worldwide annual increase is estimated to be around 3% (IDF, 2009). The overall annual increase in Europe in the age group 0–14 years from 1989 to 2003 has been 3.9%, with a higher rise in countries with a previously low incidence and having a rapid increase in standard of living (Patterson *et al.*, 2009). The increase is highest in the youngest age group, 0–5 years, at 5.4%. However, in Sweden the incidence in the age group 15–34 years is decreasing (Pundziute-Lyckå *et al.*, 2002), which suggests that the same individuals are acquiring diabetes at an earlier age. The same trend of a continuing rise in the number of new cases in the age group 0–14 years over the last 20 years has been found in the United Kingdom (around 6% per year), but not for young adults aged 15–29 years (Feltbower *et al.*, 2003).

Migration and change in incidence

There is a lack of evidence about why there is such a difference in the incidence of diabetes from one country to another, but it seems that it depends at least partly on cultural and environmental differences. For example, diabetes is more common among Asian immigrants living in the United Kingdom than in their relatives remaining in their countries of origin (Bodansky *et al.*, 1992). A possible reason for the increase in type 2 diabetes in young people may be that some people were 'programmed' thousands of years ago to survive famine by conserving energy, compared with periods when there was better access to food (Rosenbloom, 2000). Today, when we have easy access to food, these 'survival capacities' may cause problems instead. For example, the number of young people with type 2 diabetes is much higher in African Americans than among Africans still living in their home continent, although the genetic make-up of these two groups is very similar. This suggests that lifestyle and diet may be particularly important (Willi, 2000).

DIABETES HEREDITY

Although it is believed that half the factors contributing to diabetes are inherited, only 13% of children and adolescents who develop diabetes have a parent or sibling with diabetes (Willi, 2000). The risk of developing diabetes by the age of 30 for first-degree relatives (brother/sister or parent/child) is between 3% and 10% (Nordwall *et al.*, 2004). Of children with newly diagnosed diabetes, 2%–3% have a mother with type 1 diabetes, 5%–6% have a father with type 1 diabetes, and 4%–5% have a brother or sister with type 1 diabetes (Willi, 2000). In this study, only 1.5% had a first-degree relative with type 2 diabetes. Studies in identical twins have found that the risk of the other twin developing diabetes can be as high as 50%–70% (Astrup *et al.*, 2005; DCCT, 1994).

Managing diabetes during pregnancy is extremely demanding. Despite this, most mothers are strongly motivated and manage to have near-normal HbA$_{1c}$ values throughout their pregnancies. In a Scottish study, half of the women attained an HbA$_{1c}$ in the non-diabetic range at some point during their pregnancy (Rewers *et al.*, 2009). However, within 1 year, most of them increased in HbA$_{1c}$ to levels observed before pregnancy. One possible explanation for this is that the mothers had less time to take care of their diabetes in the most effective way once they had to care for their babies at home. This hypothesis is supported by research findings that women who gave birth to their second or third child had higher HbA$_{1c}$ during pregnancy, suggesting that the increased demands of childcare can impact on diabetes care during pregnancy.

Many parents who have diabetes worry that their children will also develop the condition. In one study (Gerstl *et al.*, 2008), 3% of the children of mothers with diabetes acquired diabetes by the age of 10–13 years, which is about 10 times the risk of the child of a mother without diabetes. It appears that the risk for a child of acquiring diabetes decreases as the mother's age increases. If a mother has diabetes and is older than 25 when she gives birth, the risk to the child of developing diabetes later in life is not significantly increased compared with mothers without diabetes (Boman *et al.*, 2004). Another study (Ogle, 2008) showed that 8.9% of children born to fathers with diabetes, but only 3.4% of children born to mothers with diabetes, developed the disease before the age of 20. If the mother had been 8 years old or younger when she developed diabetes, the risk to the child was considerably higher, at 13.9%. When one or both parents have diabetes, there is often a high degree of guilt if their children are diagnosed with diabetes.

LONG-TERM COMPLICATIONS

Although the prognosis of diabetes improves with each decade (Astrup *et al.*, 2005; Nordwall *et al.*, 2004), there is still a considerable risk for long-term diabetes complications. At some point following diagnosis, parents, children and young people will become aware of the long-term complications of diabetes. These include two forms of vascular disease: microvascular and macrovascular.

Microvascular disease causes retinopathy, nephropathy and neuropathy (which increases the risk of foot ulcers and sexual dysfunction). Most people will develop microvascular complications after 15–20 years of poorly controlled diabetes. According to the Department of Health (DoH, 2001, p. 2), 'diabetes is the leading cause of blindness in people of working age, the largest single cause of end stage renal failure, and excluding accidents, the biggest cause of lower limb amputation'.

Macrovascular disease causes heart disease and stroke. Heart disease is responsible for around half of all diabetes-related deaths in developed countries. There is also evidence that chronic hyperglycaemia (particularly in young boys) could be related to poorer neurocognitive outcomes (*see* Chapter 5). Evidence from the Diabetes Control and Complications Trial (DCCT, 1994) and its long-term follow-up study, Epidemiology of Diabetes Interventions and Complications (EDIC), has shown that a period of poor control can cause lasting damage – the 'metabolic memory' syndrome – even if control later improves. Therefore, it is important to aim at good control from diagnosis. A lower HbA$_{1c}$ decreases risk but does not remove it completely (DCCT, 1994).

The target HbA$_{1c}$ in all age groups has been set at < 7.5% (58 mmol/mol) by the International Society for Pediatric and Adolescent Diabetes (ISPAD, 2000; Rewers *et al.*, 2009). In a recent German-Austrian study, 58% of patients had HbA$_{1c}$ values > 7.5%, and 23% had HbA$_{1c}$ values > 9.0% (Gerstl *et al.*, 2008).

Besides the daily tasks of living with diabetes, parents often worry whether they are doing enough to prevent long-term complications. Boman and colleagues (2004) found that levels of distress in parents of children who were older that 5 years and with diabetes matched levels of those of parents of children with cancer. Both groups reported equivalent levels of uncertainty, loss of control, loss of self-esteem, disease-related fear and sleep disturbances.

THE GLOBAL PERSPECTIVE

In 2007, the total child population (between 0 and 14 years) of the world was estimated to be 1.9 billion, of whom 0.025% had diabetes. This means that approximately 480 000 children around the world have diabetes, with 76 000 new cases diagnosed each year. Around 24% come from the Southeast Asian region, but the European region, where the most reliable and up-to-date estimates of incidence are available, comes a close second, with 23% (IDF, 2009).

Lack of resources

Children and young people with diabetes need adequate amounts of insulin to survive and for them to live a full life without restrictions or disabling complications and without being stigmatised for their diabetes. It is estimated that around 70 000 children lack adequate amounts of insulin because of poverty

(Ogle, 2008). Life for a Child (www.lifeforachild.org) and Changing Diabetes in Children (www.changingdiabetesaccess.com) are two initiatives to provide these children with adequate care.

Insulin is not an expensive drug for developed countries, and most of these countries provide insulin for free to children with diabetes. However, in many developing countries insulin is expensive in relation to the total healthcare budget and it has to compete with other drugs, mainly for HIV/AIDS. There is also a high cost for blood glucose meters for self-monitoring, HbA_{1c} and the training of diabetes healthcare professionals. Beran and colleagues (2008) calculated that in Bamako, the capital of Mali, a basic minimal monthly diabetes regimen would require one blood glucose measurement, eight syringes, one vial of insulin (with an average cost of US$10.88 in the public sector) plus one monthly consultation and travel costs. It was estimated that this would come to $21.24, which corresponds to nearly 70% of the average monthly income of a Bamako citizen.

Lack of insulin as cause of death

From a global perspective, even today, almost a century after the discovery of insulin, the most common cause of death in a child with diabetes is lack of access to insulin (Gale, 2006). Field data suggest that the incidence of childhood diabetes in some countries (especially in Africa) is underestimated (Ogle, 2008), as many children die before their diabetes is diagnosed. The life expectancy of a child with newly diagnosed type 1 diabetes in rural Mozambique has been estimated to be as short as 7 months, compared with 4 years in the capital (Beran *et al.*, 2005). For Zambia, with a higher prevalence of 12 per 100 000 population, the chances are far better, but still there is only 9 years' life expectancy in rural areas and 18 years, in the capital (Beran *et al.*, 2005).

SUMMARY

Although type 1 diabetes is by far the most common type in childhood, there are many other types of diabetes that affect a smaller number of children. With increasing levels of obesity, the numbers of type 2 diabetes in adolescents have increased dramatically in some countries, especially among ethnic minority populations. There are also more rare forms of diabetes, such as monogenic diabetes. From a psychosocial perspective, both the type of diabetes and the child's family, cultural and social circumstances have a huge impact on how the child's diabetes is experienced, as well as determining the challenges the family has to face. Those families who live in poorer countries or who do not have access to resources may have to choose between saving the life of one child by buying insulin or saving the other children in the family by buying food for them. Irrespective of where they live in the world, a family living with diabetes also has to live with a heavy burden of responsibility that is relentless, and this creates a significant psychosocial strain. Worry about long-term complications may also be dependent on how well the family can cope with diabetes in the long term, leading to additional stress within the family. Parents who have diabetes themselves worry that their children will develop diabetes, and for monogenic diabetes there is an increased burden of knowing that the risk

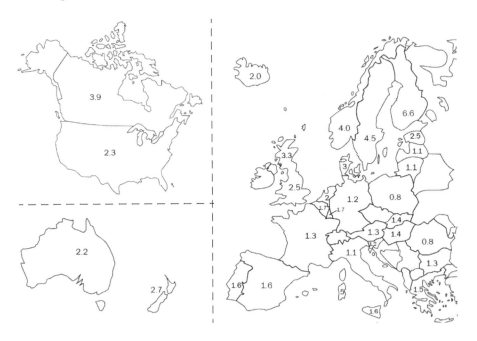

of having their children develop the same type of diabetes is as high as 50%, which adds to the stress when thinking about the future. As healthcare professionals, we have to address these needs and try to make diabetes a little bit easier to live with.

FIGURE 1.1 Approximate number of children in 1000 who will develop diabetes before the age of 15. Adapted from Green and Patterson, 2001; Karvonen *et al.*, 2000; Hanas, 2010, printed with permission.

REFERENCES

American Diabetes Association (ADA). Diagnosis and classification of diabetes mellitus. *Diabetes Care.* 2010; **33**(Suppl. 1): S62–9.

Astrup AS, Tarnow L, Rossing P, *et al.* Improved prognosis in type 1 diabetic patients with nephropathy: a prospective follow-up study. *Kidney Int.* 2005; **68**(3): 1250–7.

Beran D, McCabe A, Yudkin JS. Access to medicines versus access to treatment: the case of type 1 diabetes. *Bull World Health Organ.* 2008; **86**(8): 648–9.

Beran D, Yudkin JS, de Courten M. Access to care for patients with insulin-requiring diabetes in developing countries: case studies of Mozambique and Zambia. *Diabetes Care.* 2005; **28**(9): 2136–40.

Bodansky HJ, Staines A, Stephenson C, *et al.* Evidence for an environmental effect in the aetiology of insulin dependent diabetes in a transmigratory population. *BMJ.* 1992; **304**(6833): 1020–2.

Boman KK, Viksten J, Kogner P, *et al.* Serious illness in childhood: the different threats of cancer and diabetes from a parent perspective. *J Pediatr.* 2004; **145**(3): 373–9.

Bradley C, editor. *Handbook of Psychology and Diabetes.* Chur: Harwood Academic Publishers; 1994.

Burdick J, Chase HP, Slover RH, *et al.* Missed insulin meal boluses and elevated hemoglobin A1c levels in children receiving insulin pump therapy. *Pediatrics.* 2004; **113**(3 Pt. 1): e221–4.

Craig ME, Hattersley A, Donaghue KC. Definition, epidemiology and classification of diabetes in children and adolescents. *Pediatr Diabetes.* 2009; **10**(Suppl. 12): 3–12.

Department of Health (DoH). *Diabetes Service Framework for Diabetes: standards.* London: DoH publications; 2001.

Diabetes Control and Complications Trial Research Group (DCCT). Effect of intensive diabetes treatment on the development and progression of long-term complications in adolescents with insulin-dependent diabetes mellitus: Diabetes Control and Complications Trial. *J Pediatr.* 1994; **125**(2): 177–88.

Diglas J, Feinböck C, Winkler F, *et al.* Reduced pain perception with an automatic injection device for use with an insulin pen. *Horm Res.* 1998; **50**: A30.

Ehtisham S, Barrett TG, Shaw NJ. Type 2 diabetes mellitus in UK children: an emerging problem. *Diabet Med.* 2000; **17**(12): 867–71.

Feltbower RG, McKinney PA, Parslow RC, *et al.* Type 1 diabetes in Yorkshire, UK: time trends in 0–14 and 15–29-year-olds, age at onset and age-period-cohort modelling. *Diabet Med.* 2003; **20**(6): 437–41.

Gale EA. Dying of diabetes. *Lancet.* 2006; **368**(9548): 1626–8.

Gerstl EM, Rabl W, Rosenbauer J, *et al.* Metabolic control as reflected by HbA1c in children, adolescents and young adults with type-1 diabetes mellitus: combined longitudinal analysis including 27,035 patients from 207 centers in Germany and Austria during the last decade. *Eur J Pediatr.* 2008; **167**(4): 447–53.

Graff MR, McClanahan MA. Assessment by patients with diabetes mellitus of two insulin pen delivery systems versus a vial and syringe. *Clin Ther.* 1998; **20**(3): 486–96.

Green A, Patterson CC, EURODIAB TIGER Study Group. Trends in the incidence of childhood-onset diabetes in Europe 1989–1998. *Diabetologia.* 2001; **44**(Suppl. 3): B3–8.

Hanas R. *Type 1 Diabetes in Children, Adolescents and Young Adults.* London: Class Health; 2010.

Hanas R, Adolfsson P, Elfvin-Akesson K, *et al.* Indwelling catheters used from the onset of diabetes decrease injection pain and pre-injection anxiety. *J Pediatr.* 2002; **140**(3): 315–20.

Hanas R, Ludvigsson J. Experience of pain from insulin injections and needle-phobia in young patients with IDDM. *Pract Diab Int.* 1997; **14**(4): 95–9.

Harjutsalo V, Sjöberg L, Tuomilehto J. Time trends in the incidence of type 1 diabetes in Finnish children: a cohort study. *Lancet.* 2008; **371**(9626): 1777–82.

Hattersley AT, Ashcroft FM. Activating mutations in Kir6.2 and neonatal diabetes: new clinical syndromes, new scientific insights, and new therapy. *Diabetes.* 2005; **54**(9): 2503–13.

Hattersley A, Bruining J, Shield J, *et al.* The diagnosis and management of monogenic diabetes in children and adolescents. *Pediatr Diabetes.* 2009; **10**(Suppl. 12): 33–42.

International Diabetes Foundation (IDF). Diabetes in the young: a global perspective. *Diabetes Atlas.* 2009; **3**: 2027–33.

International Society for Pediatric and Adolescent Diabetes (ISPAD). *Consensus Guidelines for the Management of Type 1 Diabetes Mellitus in Children and Adolescents.* 2011. Available at: www.ispad.org/NewsFiles/IDF-ISPAD_Diabetes_in_Childhood_and%20 Adolescence_Guidelines_2011.pdf

Jefferson IG, Swift PG, Skinner TC, *et al.* Diabetes services in the UK: third national survey confirms continuing deficiencies. *Arch Dis Child.* 2003; **88**(1): 53–6.

Karvonen M, Viik-Kajander M, Moltchanova E, *et al.* Incidence of childhood type 1 diabetes worldwide: Diabetes Mondiale (DiaMond) Project Group. *Diabetes Care.* 2000; **23**(10): 1516–26.

Klingensmith G, Kaufman F, Schatz D, *et al.* Care of children with diabetes in the school and day care setting. *Diabetes Care.* 2003; **26**(Suppl. 1): S131–5.

Liese AD, D'Agostino RB Jr, Hamman RF, *et al.* The burden of diabetes mellitus among US youth: prevalence estimates from the SEARCH for Diabetes in Youth Study. *Pediatrics.* 2006; **118**(4): 1510–18.

Lteif AN, Schwenk WF. Accuracy of pen injectors versus insulin syringes in children with type 1 diabetes. *Diabetes Care.* 1999; **22**(1): 137–40.

Nordwall M, Bojestig M, Arnqvist HJ, *et al.* Declining incidence of severe retinopathy and persisting decrease of nephropathy in an unselected population of type 1 diabetes: the Linköping Diabetes Complications Study. *Diabetologia.* 2004; **47**(7): 1266–72.

Ogle G. Children with diabetes in the developing world. *Pract Diab Int.* 2008; **25**: 351–2.

O'Riordan SM, Robinson PD, Donaghue KC, *et al.* Management of cystic fibrosis-related diabetes in children and adolescents. *Pediatr Diabetes.* 2009; **10**(Suppl. 12): 43–50.

Patterson CC, Dahlquist GG, Gyürüs E, *et al.* Incidence trends for childhood type 1 diabetes in Europe during 1989–2003 and predicted new cases 2005–20: a multicentre prospective registration study. *Lancet.* 2009; **373**(9680): 2027–33.

Peyrot M, Aanstoot H. Parent-reported social, psychological, and health care factors associated with youth self-care success in the Multi-national DAWN Youth Survey. *Pediatr Diabetes.* 2008; **9**(Suppl. 10): 28–35.

Phillip M, Battelino T, Rodriguez H, *et al.* Use of insulin pump therapy in the pediatric age-group: consensus statement from the European Society for Paediatric Endocrinology, the Lawson Wilkins Pediatric Endocrine Society, and the International Society for Pediatric and Adolescent Diabetes, endorsed by the American Diabetes Association and the European Association for the Study of Diabetes. *Diabetes Care.* 2007; **30**(6): 1653–62.

Pundziute-Lyckå A, Dahlquist G, Nyström L, *et al.* The incidence of type I diabetes has not increased but shifted to a younger age at diagnosis in the 0–34 years group in Sweden 1983–1998. *Diabetologia.* 2002; **45**(6): 783–91.

Rewers M, Pihoker C, Donaghue K, *et al.* Assessment and monitoring of glycemic control in children and adolescents with diabetes. *Pediatr Diabetes.* 2009; **10**(Suppl. 12): 71–81.

Rosenbloom A. The cause of the epidemic of type 2 diabetes in children. *Curr Opin Endocrinol Diabetes.* 2000; **7**(4): 191–6.

Särnblad S, Berg L, Detlofsson I, *et al.* Diabetes care in Swedish schools: a national survey. *Pediatric Diabetes.* 2009; **10**(Suppl. 11): 1–1–9.

Skogsberg L, Fors H, Hanas R, *et al.* Improved treatment satisfaction but no difference in metabolic control when using continuous subcutaneous insulin infusion vs. multiple daily injections in children at onset of type 1 diabetes mellitus. *Pediatr Diabetes.* 2008; **9**(5): 472–9.

Slingerland AS, Shields BM, Flanagan SE, *et al.* Referral rates for diagnostic testing support an incidence of permanent neonatal diabetes in three European countries of at least 1 in 260,000 live births. *Diabetologia.* 2009; **52**(8): 1683–5.

Sullivan-Bolyai S, Knafl K, Tamborlane W, *et al.* Parents' reflections on managing their children's diabetes with insulin pumps. *J Nurs Scholarsh.* 2004; **36**(4): 316–23.

Tattersall R, Travis B. *Treatment of Insulin-Dependent Diabetes: art or science* [lecture]. Stockholm; 1993.

Weissberg-Benchell J, Goodman SS, Antisdel Lomaglio J, *et al.* The use of continuous subcutaneous insulin infusion (CSII): parental and professional perceptions of self-care mastery and autonomy in children and adolescents. *J Pediatr Psychol.* 2007; **32**(10): 1196–202.

Willi SM. Type 2 diabetes mellitus in adolescents. *Curr Opin Endocrinol Diabetes.* 2000; **7**(2): 71–6.

World Health Organization (WHO). *Definition, Diagnosis and Classification of Diabetes Mellitus and its Complications. Part 1: Diagnosis and Classification of Diabetes Mellitus.* Geneva: WHO/NCD/NCS/99.2; 1999.

Wysocki T, Meinhold PM, Taylor A, *et al.* Psychometric properties and normative data for the parent version of the diabetes independence survey. *Diabetes Educ.* 1996; **22**(6): 587–91.

CHAPTER 2

The impact of diagnosis

Clarissa Martin, Julia Núñez and Daniel Royo

INTRODUCTION

Diabetes is a life-threatening condition, and its diagnosis has a profound psychological impact on both the child and the parents. Acute psychological distress may decrease – but not disappear – in the 12 months following diagnosis. Research suggests that children and young people with diabetes are at risk of adjustment problems during the initial period of adaptation after diagnosis and are at higher risk of continued adjustment difficulties and mental health problems thereafter (e.g. Grey *et al.*, 1998; Kovacks *et al.*, 1997; Lloyd, 2010). Their families often experience loss and unresolved grief, which may cause further psychological problems, such as chronic sorrow and depression. Life-related stress factors, such as family conflict, financial difficulties or marital problems, are also associated with poorer metabolic control.

This chapter describes the impact a diagnosis of diabetes can have for children, young people, their parents and the family as a whole. It considers the different stages of development from early childhood to adolescence and how the diagnosis may be experienced at each of these stages. The ensuing psychological consequences for the child and family are also described.

RECEIVING THE DIAGNOSIS OF DIABETES: A RIPPLE EFFECT

There is agreement within both the research literature and clinical practice that receiving a diagnosis of diabetes is experienced as a life-changing event. Parkes's theory of psychosocial transition (Parkes, 1971) argues that life-changing events require people to undertake a major revision of their assumptions of the world in order to adapt themselves to the new situation. People facing a life-changing event undergo a 'psychosocial transition', requiring them to learn new cognitions, emotions and patterns of behaviours that will allow them to continue to develop and survive. Transitions are required when a sudden or planned event produces vital changes within a person's life (Spierer, 1977). This results in a transformation in the relationships that individuals maintain with their environment (Schlossberg, 1995). Hopson *et al.* (1992) identified the key emotions and feelings experienced within transition times and developed a model to help understand this pattern (*see* Box 2.1).

BOX 2.1 Seven Transition Stages Model (Hopson *et al.*, 1992)

- Shock: the awareness of emotions appears blocked.
- Denial: the importance of the change is minimised.
- Self-doubt and depression: experience of uncertainty and doubts related to how to control the new situation.
- Acceptance of the new reality: the acceptance of the new reality starts with detachment from the old patterns.
- Analysis of the possibilities for resolution: at this stage, individuals start to take a more active role through trying new coping strategies.
- Looking for meaning: the need for understanding; how the individual's future will be affected is developed.
- Integration: the new experience is fully incorporated and integrated within the individual's life.

The relevance of this theory to adjustment of diagnosis of childhood diabetes has not been extensively researched. However, the concept of 'transition' is congruent with responses of parents to the loss of their 'healthy child' and fits with the grieving and adaptation processes that many seem to experience. Children and young people diagnosed with diabetes and their families have to change established behaviours (e.g. the freedom to eat sweets at any time) and to develop new behaviours that allow them to adapt to the new situation (such as learning to inject insulin). A diagnosis of diabetes may trigger initial feelings of fear, uncertainty and distrust when diabetes is still unknown territory, and further emotions may develop through the different stages of adaptation to the illness. Northam *et al.* (1996) found that the emotional reaction to the hospitalisation experience, the 'loss of a healthy identity' and the fact that a restrictive and painful treatment must be accepted was very intense at the moment of diagnosis in children between 1 and 14 years of age and their families.

Psychological consequences of the diagnosis

Guidelines of the International Society for Pediatric and Adolescent Diabetes state that psychosocial factors are the most important influences affecting the care and management of diabetes (ISPAD, 2000). This is based on a literature that has clearly demonstrated a relationship between living with diabetes and emotional and behavioural difficulties. For example, Kovacs *et al.* (1985) investigated children from their diagnosis until they were 10 years of age. They found that half of the children studied had been diagnosed with a psychiatric disorder (usually anxiety and depression) and that females with poor glycaemic control had a greater probability of being diagnosed with mental health problems. In a subsequent study (Kovacs *et al.*, 1990), they found that almost two thirds of children with diabetes showed mild symptoms of sadness and felt socially isolated. Anxiety and low self-esteem have also been associated with poor metabolic control (Anderson *et al.*, 1981) and a relationship among poor psychological adjustment, anxiety symptoms and negative mood has been reported (Close *et al.*, 1986; Fonagy *et al.*, 1987; Grey *et al.*, 2002). These studies suggest that a diagnosis of diabetes may have far-reaching implications for the child.

It is not surprising that parents experience stress, depression and anxiety as a consequence of their child's diagnosis. While some research argues that adjustment-related psychological problems in parents are resolved after the first year of receiving the diagnosis (Delamater, 2000, 2007), other studies find that feelings of grief continue for up to 7 years post-diagnosis (Lowes and Lyne, 2000).

Case study 1: Eva's mother

I separated from my husband the year after my only daughter, Eva, was diagnosed with diabetes, just after her 10th birthday. Six months after her diagnosis, Eva become more able to manage her diabetes independently, but she started to be careless with meals, would skip insulin injections and ignore blood glucose measures. I had suffered depression when I was younger and had taken medication that worked well. However, this time I felt depressed and ended up in the hospital. Eva moved in with her father until I recovered. My physical recuperation was quicker than the psychological one. It took me a long time to recover my emotional stability. I felt guilty and unable as a mother to protect my child and to take care of her diabetes. After several months of therapy with the psychologist, I started to feel better. I met people in the same circumstances as me. A couple with two daughters were living near my house. Their youngest girl was diabetic and the same age as Eva. They helped me a lot and we become very good friends. I had somebody I could rely on to help with Eva's diabetes. Eva came back to live with me when her father found a job.

At the time of the diagnosis, families have to accommodate the new situation and demonstrate an ability to manage the practical requirements and complexities of diabetes control. Readjustment of the family dynamics is needed to manage the diabetes, while at the same time balancing the quality of life of the child affected – as well as the needs of the rest of the family members (Riekert and Drotar, 1999). In some families, the diagnosis can act as a trigger for the emergence of pre-existing psychological, behavioural or family problems. The assumption of responsibility, shared by the parents in different degrees, may also generate guilty feelings, frustration or fear. It is common for the primary responsibility for care and decision-making to be taken on by mothers, which may also be a cause of stress within the family system.

CHILDREN AND THEIR FAMILIES DEALING WITH THE DIAGNOSIS
Preschool children (between 0 and 5 years)
Early childhood is a period of extraordinary change. Between birth and the third year of life, the majority of children double their height and weight, growing in stature and progressing towards more adult-like physical characteristics. The newborn reflexes disappear within the first year of life and motor development increases. By the age of three, children have mastered many motor skills, such as walking, using utensils, catching a ball and so forth; by the age of five, they can balance on one foot and they have fine motor skills using pencils and scissors. These physical and motor changes run parallel with social skills, language and cognitive development.

Socio-emotional skills are also developed from the age of 3–5 years. Social skills include the formation of peer relationships, gender identification and the development of a sense of right and wrong. Expressive language, beginning typically around the first year, increases considerably in the middle of the second year, and by year five it is usually well developed, with all of the 'building blocks' of adult language in place. As their language skills develop, children start using symbols and thinking about 'here and now' situations.

At this stage of development, children are still focused on the present and have difficulties conceptualising time and using logical thinking. As a result, children under the age of 5 years are unable to fully understand the future implications of their condition. The different aspects of handling diabetes can result in difficulties between the toddler and the parents affecting the parent–child relationship (Wysocki et al., 1989). Ensuring rigid, timetabled routines in relation to meals and insulin injections can be a challenge in a stage of development marked by rapidly changing preferences in relation to food. Furthermore, the level of cognitive ability in this age group means they may experience the treatment as invasive, which can result in aggression, anxiety or refusal to allow injections or blood tests to be carried out. This can cause difficulties at mealtimes.

BOX 2.2 Frequent challenges for parents of preschoolers (Leaverton, 1979)

- Glycaemic control.
- The implementation of a regular meal schedule. (This aspect has been improved by the use of longer-acting insulin that allows greater flexibility around mealtimes.)
- The lack of understanding by the child with regard to the insulin injections.
- Sibling rivalry due to the increased attention the child with diabetes receives.
- The greater risk of severe hypoglycaemia in children under 5 years old due to the fact that children at this stage cannot fully communicate their needs.
- Irregularity of physical exercise.

Vandagriff *et al.* (1992) found that parents of preschool children with diabetes worried more than those of older children with diabetes, although the level of worry did not correlate with the degree of diabetes control. One of the major concerns of parents of preschool children with diabetes is the fear of their child suffering hypoglycaemia, especially at night while the child is asleep (*see* Chapter 3). In clinical practice, it is common to find that parents repeatedly check glucose levels during the night, as well as making routine visits to the child's bedroom. Studies have indicated that toddlers with diabetes are at a particularly high risk of suffering neurological deterioration–related hypoglycaemia (e.g. Rovet *et al.*, 1987; Northam *et al.*, 1996). Health professionals can recommend continuous glucose metres that will set off an alarm at low glucose levels in order to help reduce parental anxiety. The need for medical guidance alongside continuing education and psychosocial support for families of preschool children with diabetes has been highlighted in the literature (e.g. Golden *et al.*, 1985).

Case study 2: Julian's mother

Julian was 15 months old when he started crying continuously and was always thirsty. We took him to the doctor several times, but gastroenteritis was suggested. One morning, he started vomiting and convulsing and his eyes had a strange look. We took him to the nearest hospital emergency department. He was diagnosed with diabetes type 1 and had diabetic ketoacidosis (DKA). He was in the intensive care unit for 2 days, and afterwards he was kept on the hospital ward for further treatment. I was in hospital with him for 8 days, and it was there that I started to understand all the different aspects of diabetes and its treatment. I personally have experienced how living with diabetes can put families under considerable strain. I had to learn how to administer insulin injections and overcome my phobia of needles, learn about the symptoms of DKA and how to do a sugar test, manage Julian's diet so he could get the right kind of food at the right time and learn about lifestyle – things like how important it was to exercise. I knew that this was going to cause a big change in our family lifestyle. Suddenly, diabetes was a kind of 'guest' living in our family without ever having been invited!

Children between 6 and 12 years old

As children get older, physical growth slows down in comparison to earlier stages. Body proportions and motor skills are established at this point and become more refined. From a cognitive perspective, this is the stage where children develop the ability to think logically and in abstract terms. They also develop socially through the expanded social context at school. They learn to take other people's perspectives and to develop friendships with peers. By the time they are around 9 years old, they can tell stories and describe characters from authors' perspectives, as well as expressing their own opinions.

At this stage of development, children have the ability to make relationships with peers and are aware of the social consequences of their behaviour. As a result of this, they may exhibit more self-control and may develop a more active role towards the challenges of living with diabetes. Families can sometimes react to this negatively, becoming overprotective and limiting the child's ability to begin to manage their treatment. Conversely, the development of social interactions can be adversely affected by diabetes where there is poor metabolic control, which can lead to withdrawal and isolation.

School-age children may also experience anxiety on returning to school post-diagnosis, as they may feel 'different' from their peers. They will need time and space to carry out blood glucose testing and insulin injections. A school plan should clearly identify and agree a protocol for the management of hypoglycaemia. Nabors et al. (2008) reported that up to 61% of parents believed that their children needed the constant supervision of an adult for the appropriate control of the illness during school hours. In contrast, Bradbury and Smith (1983) showed that only 25% of teachers had appropriate knowledge of diabetes, with an even smaller percentage admitting knowing what to do in a diabetes-related emergency. Teachers and fellow students should be educated in diabetes with the goal of eliminating myths and prejudices.

At this stage of development, early detection and treatment of emotional or behavioural difficulties are essential. Kovacs et al. (1997) reported that difficulty with initial adjustment was a predictor of future anxiety. Two years after diagnosis, children with diabetes continue to show higher levels of dependency, depression and isolation (Grey and Boland, 1996).

Case study 3: Jonathan's parents

Jonathan was 8 years old when the symptoms of diabetes type 1 began. He was always thirsty and tired, and in 1 month lost 9 kg. He spent 3 days in the hospital intensive care unit and a further month on the hospital ward. When he came home, he rebelled against the treatment regime, and we were constantly in fear of him suffering hypoglycaemia. We were always scared of hypoglycaemia – mainly at night. I thought that giving him more freedom was a bad idea because his diabetes management could get out of control. I was worried sick. But we found that his behaviour improved when we sent him to a holiday camp for children with diabetes. He witnessed children younger than himself giving themselves insulin shots . . . and he decided to inject by himself. He also made new friends and was able to maintain the contact through email. One of these new friends was living in our neighbourhood, so we also made friends with his family. Since then, we have supported each other.

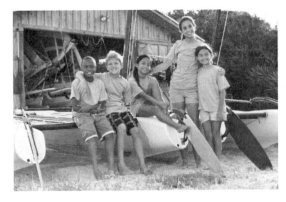

Diabetes summer camp: an opportunity for the development of new self-confidence

Adolescents (from 13 to 18 years old)

Adolescence is a period of intense physical, psychological and social change. During this time, young people are creating a stable identity and gender-related roles, building mature relationships with peers and achieving emotional independence as they become mature adults. The diagnosis of diabetes can clash with the natural completion of these tasks, creating anxiety and stress.

Equally, the developmental tasks may interfere with the self-management behaviour required for adequate diabetes control. Younger adolescents who are still focused on the present may dismiss the long-term potential complications of diabetes (Hanna and Guthrie, 2000). They also may experience their parents' concerns about everyday diabetes tasks as less important than peer relationships and social activities (Allen *et al.*, 1984), or they may try high-risk behaviours – such as drinking – in an attempt to control their environment, resulting in poor adherence and metabolic control (Grey *et al.*, 1998).

There is no agreement in the literature about the appropriate age for independent self-management of diabetes (Johnson, 1995). However, self-management imposed too early has been associated with poorer psychological adjustment and glycaemic control (Ingersoll *et al.*, 1986; La Greca, 1990).

A few studies have evaluated gender differences in relationship to glycaemic control. Naar-King *et al.* (2006) found that boys were less likely to express themselves and had a tendency to externalise their symptoms. The research suggested that this behaviour impacted negatively in their communication with the doctors caring for them. As a consequence, they had a worse relationship with their doctors than girls (Bearman and La Greca, 2002; Grey *et al.*, 1997). Other authors (e.g. Perwien *et al.*, 2000) describe a positive relationship between abilities to achieve metabolic control and female gender, suggesting males are in need of closer supervision than females. Given the small number of studies in this area, results have to be considered with caution.

Case study 4: Maria's experience of the diagnosis

I was 16 when I started to suffer nausea, vomiting and loss of appetite. I really felt very tired. My parents were alarmed by my excessive weight loss. My symptoms were initially blamed on anorexia. One day, I could not even get out of bed and was vomiting constantly, so my mother called an ambulance. A few minutes later, an ambulance and a doctor arrived at my house. My mother explained the symptoms to the doctor and he took out a machine that I had never seen before and pricked my finger. I did not understand what was going on, because diabetes was a new concept to me. I thought that it would be nothing serious; perhaps a simple treatment and I would return home immediately. However, I was taken to the intensive care unit, where I was admitted and stayed for 3 days due to diabetic ketoacidosis. This experience was a dividing line for me – a split in time between before and after the diagnosis – because I had to face the irreversibility of the disease and its consequences. Since the diagnosis, I have suffered from anxiety, which I put down to all the problems I have with diabetes.

Psychological consequences of the diagnosis in adolescents

The challenges that the diagnosis of diabetes present to adolescent emotional well-being are covered in detail in Chapter 3. Research has shown that the incidence of mental health problems is higher in young people with diabetes (Northam, 2004). For example, De Groot and Lustman (2001) found that depression was twice as frequent in patients with diabetes than in healthy controls. Depression has also been associated with poor glycaemic control and increased hospitalisations in adolescents (La Greca *et al.*, 1995). Kovacks *et al.* (1990) stated that depressive symptoms related to diabetes increased after the first year of diagnosis, while anxiety decreased. However, self-esteem was a stable feature, independent of the level of metabolic control. There is also evidence that adolescents with diabetes, especially females, have a higher incidence of eating disorders (*see* Chapter 13) than their non-diabetic counterparts and that this is associated with poor glycaemic control (Jones *et al.*, 2000). Close *et al.* (1986) found that 28% of adolescents with diabetes also have concurrent behavioural or emotional difficulties and 12% of their parents also experience depressive symptoms.

THE CONSEQUENCES OF DIAGNOSIS ON FAMILY FUNCTIONING

The impact of the diagnosis in family interactions shows different patterns that vary with the age and stage of development of the individual diagnosed, as well as those of the different family members (Delamater, 2007). Diabetes affects the emotional well-being and behaviour of the whole family, not just the diagnosed individual (Rubin and Peyrot, 1992). Communication patterns, interaction styles and alliances within the family network can be altered as the family adapts to the physical and psychological demands of a complex and severe illness (Cerreto and Travis, 1984). Furthermore, parents of children and young people with diabetes may feel that diabetes is threatening the stability of the family unit. These worries can result in all family members mobilising to protect their position within the family system. Subsystem boundaries, such as those among siblings, may become weakened and easily crossed. As a result, family hierarchies can also become affected, with siblings adopting parental roles in the absence of an effective parental subsystem. For example, a younger brother or sister may take on caring for an older brother or sister with diabetes.

Case study 5: Noel's mother's experience

Five months after Noel was diagnosed with diabetes, his father and I separated. He left the home, and from that moment I became a single mother of three children. We'd had several crises during our marriage, but diabetes was the last straw. We disagreed constantly on how to help Noel manage his diabetes. His father wanted his only boy to be tough and accused me of being an overprotective and controlling mother. I thought that it was just too much pressure for a 7-year-old boy. I knew that Noel was going to be my last baby, and I suppose this was the way I saw him. However, I was the one looking after him when he was admitted to hospital with diabetic ketoacidosis. At the beginning, my ex-husband came every day to visit him, but from the second week he just telephoned to see how he was doing. I felt he couldn't cope with seeing his son so ill, but he wouldn't admit to having any feelings about the situation because he thought that made him weak. My oldest daughter had to look after her sister while I was at the hospital. I thought it was too much for her because she had to stop going out with her friends, cook for both of them, clean the house and so on. My mother was a widow, and so she moved in with us to help me. It took a long time for me to recover from this experience.

According to Wolfsdorf *et al.* (1994), a common error of health professionals is the overwhelming amount of information given to parents at a time when they are still affected by the initial shock. Golden *et al.* (1985) highlighted the importance of providing psychosocial and educational support to families in conjunction with medical visits. The emotional stress that families may experience at the time of diagnosis increases as they become more aware of the long list of unavoidable daily tasks that need to be completed as part of day-to-day diabetes management.

BOX 2.3 Family emotions after diagnosis of diabetes (adapted from Hopson *et al.*, 1992)

- *Shock*: usually lasting from the moment of diagnosis until a few weeks afterwards. Common reactions are denial and confusion. As a result, the parents may experience changes in eating and sleeping habits as well as generalised anxiety. It is important to support the family in order to keep the situation from affecting them negatively, e.g. focusing attention on the child with the diagnosis to the detriment of attention given to the siblings, developing misconceptions about the illness and so forth.
- *Confrontation*: the trip home from hospital is a key moment. A reality check occurs when decisions must be made and the family still need direct support from health professionals. It is a difficult phase, and it is where family conflicts may emerge. Underlying mental health problems such as depression and/or anxiety may come to the surface.
- *Recovery*: this state usually begins a year after the diagnosis has been made.

An emotional strengthening and adjustments can be appreciated. The mourning period of the diagnosis cannot be endless; positive emotions must be highlighted by doing such things as helping others in similar situations and looking at successfully completed goals.

Lowes and Lyne (2000) argue that parents of children with diabetes deal with the tension of managing the requirements of the illness in different ways and in accordance with their interpersonal abilities. A diagnosis of diabetes means all family members have to change their behaviour patterns (Mellin *et al.*, 2004). For example, spontaneity is generally reduced and substituted with control and planning, such as having food and insulin nearby. Mellin and colleagues (2004) found that 30% of the parents in their study experienced diabetes as a family burden and 37% of them felt guilty about the diagnosis. Research has also suggested that families whose members have high levels of support achieve closer adherence to the proposed treatment.

Delamater (2000) found that the families of young people with diabetes who presented with metabolic- and adherence-related problems exhibited more relationship conflicts, more financial problems and less cohesion and stability than families where the young person had better metabolic control. Improvement in metabolic control has also been associated with better communication among the members of the families and better problem-solving ability. Overstreet *et al.* (1995) supported these findings and also described greater difficulty in managing behaviour among parents of young people with diabetes.

These shifts in the family system also have a tremendous impact on siblings, although this aspect has been less researched. In general, siblings of children with chronic conditions have been shown to be at higher risk of emotional and behavioural problems (Jackson *et al.*, 2008). As parents learn new skills and focus on the child with diabetes, siblings may feel uncared for and unimportant, angry with the brother or sister who has been diagnosed and at the same time they may feel guilty. The intention of parents may be to protect healthy siblings from unnecessary burdens. However, the consequence of this may be for siblings to feel excluded from family activities. Siblings may also adopt new roles in order to adapt to the new family dynamics. For example, they may take on the role of the 'helper' for their brother or sister with diabetes and also for their parents in dealing with medical regimens and other household duties. Some children keep a low profile so as not to 'cause further problems' and become 'invisible', while others may act out to gain attention and 'distract' the family from the illness of their sibling. These factors make it essential that health professionals and parents include siblings as part of the process of the family adjustment to the diabetes.

SUMMARY

Diabetes is a life-threatening condition that causes distress in children and young people, as well as in their families. The ultimate impact of the diagnosis depends on many internal and external factors, including the child's developmental level at the time of the diagnosis and the resources and structure of the family system. The provision of psychological support to children, young people and their families at the time of the diagnosis as well as during the later phases in the young person's life has been acknowledged as an essential component of long-term diabetes management and care.

REFERENCES

Allen DA, Affleck G, Tennen H, *et al.* Concerns of children with a chronic illness: a cognitive-developmental study of juvenile diabetes. *Child Care Health Dev.* 1984; **10**(4): 211–18.

Anderson BJ, Miller JP, Auslander WF, *et al.* Family characteristics of diabetic adolescents: relationship to metabolic control. *Diabetes Care.* 1981; **4**(6): 586–93.

Bearman KJ, La Greca AM. Assessing friend support of adolescents' diabetes care: the diabetes social support questionnaire-friends version. *J Pediatr Psychol.* 2002; **27**(5): 417–28.

Bradbury AJ, Smith CS. An assessment of the diabetic knowledge of school teachers. *Arch Dis Child.* 1983; **58**: 692–6.

Cerreto MC, Travis LB. Implications of psychological and family factors in the treatment of diabetes. *Pediatr Clin North Am.* 1984; **31**(3): 689–710.

Close H, Davies AG, Price DA, *et al.* Emotional difficulties in diabetes mellitus. *Arch Dis Child.* 1986; **61**(4): 337–40.

De Groot M, Lustman PJ. Depression among African-Americans with diabetes: a dearth of studies. *Diabetes Care.* 2001; **24**(2): 407–8.

Delamater AM. Quality of life in youths with diabetes. *Diabetes Spectrum.* 2000; **13**: 42–6.

Delamater AM. Psychological care of children and adolescents with diabetes. *Pediatr Diabetes.* 2007; **8**(5): 340–8.

Fonagy P, Moran GS, Lindsay MK, *et al.* Psychological adjustment and diabetic control. *Arch Dis Child.* 1987; **62**(10): 1009–13.

Golden MP, Russell BP, Ingerlsoll GM, *et al.* Management of diabetes mellitus in children younger than 5 years of age. *Am J Dis Child.* 1985; **139**(5): 448–52.

Grey M, Boland EA. Diabetes mellitus (type I). In: Jackson PL, Vessey JA, editors. *Primary Care of the Child with a Chronic Condition.* 2nd ed. St. Louis: Mosby-Year Book; 1996. pp. 350–70.

Grey M, Boland EA, Yu C, *et al.* Personal and family factors associated with quality of life in adolescents with diabetes. *Diabetes Care.* 1998; **21**(6): 909–14.

Grey M, Lipman T, Cameron ME, *et al.* Coping behaviors at diagnosis and in adjustment one year later in children with diabetes. *Nurs Res.* 1997; **46**(6): 312–17.

Grey M, Whittemore R, Tamborlane W. Depression in type 1 diabetes in children: natural history and correlates. *J Psychosom Res.* 2002; **53**(4): 907–11.

Hanna KM, Guthrie DW. Adolescents' perceived benefits and barriers related to diabetes self-management: part 1. *Issues Compr Pediatr Nurs.* 2000; **23**(3): 165–74.

Hopson B, Scally M, Stafford K. *Transitions: the challenge of change.* Lifeskills Personal Development Series. London: Lifeskills Communication; 1992.

Ingersoll GM, Orr DP, Herrold AJ, *et al.* Cognitive maturity and self-management among adolescents with insulin-dependent diabetes mellitus. *J Pediatr.* 1986; **108**(4): 620–3.

International Society for Pediatric and Adolescent Diabetes (ISPAD). *Consensus Guidelines for the Management of Type 1 Diabetes Mellitus in Children and Adolescents.* 2011. Available at: www.ispad.org/NewsFiles/IDF-ISPAD_Diabetes_in_Childhood_and%20 Adolescence_Guidelines_2011.pdf

Jackson C, Richer J, Edge JA. Sibling psychological adjustment to type 1 diabetes mellitus. *Pediatr Diabetes.* 2008; **9**(4): 308–11.

Johnson SB. Managing insulin-dependent diabetes mellitus in adolescence: a developmental perspective. In: Wallander JL, Siegel LJ, editors. *Adolescent Health Problems: behavioral perspectives.* New York, NY: Guilford Press; 1995. pp. 265–88.

Jones J, Lawsone M, Daneman D, *et al.* Eating disorders in adolescent females with and without type 1 diabetes: cross sectional study. *BMJ.* 2000; **310**(10): 1563–6.

Kovacs M, Feinberg TL, Paulauskas S, *et al.* Initial coping responses and psychosocial characteristics of children with insulin-dependent diabetes mellitus. *J Pediatr.* 1985; **106**(5): 827–34.

Kovacs M, Goldston D, Obrosky D, *et al.* Psychiatric disorders in youths with IDDM: rates and risk factors. *Diabetes Care.* 1997; **20**(1): 36–44.

Kovacs M, Iyengar S, Goldston D, *et al.* Psychological functioning of children with insulin-dependent diabetes mellitus: a longitudinal study. *J Pediatr Psychol.* 1990; **15**(5): 619–32.

La Greca AM. Social consequences of pediatric conditions: fertile area for future investigation and intervention? *J Pediatr Psychol.* 1990; **15**(5): 285–308.

La Greca AM, Swales T, Klemp S, *et al.* Adolescents with diabetes: gender differences in psychosocial functioning and glycemic control. *Child Health Care.* 1995; **24**: 61–78.

Leaverton DR. The child with diabetes mellitus. In: Call JD, Noshpitz JD, Berlin IN, Cohen RL *et al.*, editors. *Basic Handbook of Child Psychiatry.* Vol. 1. New York, NY: Basic Books; 1979. pp. 452–8.

Lloyd, CE. Diabetes and mental health: the problem of co-morbidity. *Diabet Med.* 2010; **27**(8): 853–4.

Lowes L, Lyne P. Chronic sorrow in parents of children with newly diagnosed diabetes: a review of the literature and discussion of the implications for nursing practice. *J Adv Nurs.* 2000; **32**(1): 41–8.

Mellin AE, Neumark-Sztainer D, Patterson J, *et al.* Unhealthy weight management behaviour among adolescent girls with type 1 diabetes mellitus: the role of familial eating patterns and weight-related concerns. *J Adolesc Health.* 2004; **35**(4): 278–89.

Naar-King S, Idalski A, Ellis D, *et al.* Gender differences in adherence and metabolic control in urban youth with poorly controlled type 1 diabetes: the mediating role of mental health symptoms. *J Pediatr Psychol.* 2006; **3**: 793–802.

Nabors LA, Little SG, Akin-Little A, *et al.* Teacher knowledge of and confidence in meeting the needs of children with chronic medical conditions: pediatric psychology's contribution to education. *Psychol Schools.* 2008; **45**(3): 217–26.

Northam E, Anderson P, Adler R, *et al.* Psychosocial and family functioning in children with insulin-dependent diabetes at diagnosis and one year later. *J Pediatr Psychol.* 1996; **21**(5): 699–717.

Northam EA, Matthews LK, Anderson PJ, *et al.* Psychiatric morbidity and health outcome in type 1 diabetes: perspectives from a prospective longitudinal study. *Diabet Med.* 2004; **22**(2): 152–7.

Overstreet S, Goins J, Chen RS, *et al.* Family environment and the interrelation of family structure, child behavior, and metabolic control for children with diabetes. *J Pediatr Psychol.*1995; **20**(4): 435–47.

Parkes CM. Psycho-social transitions: A field for study. *Soc Sci Med.*1971; **5**: 105–15.

Perwien AR, Johnson SB, Dymtrow D, *et al.* Blood glucose monitoring skills in children with type I diabetes. *Clin Pediatr (Phila).* 2000; **39**(6): 351–7.

Riekert KA, Drotar D. Who participates in research on adherence to treatment in insulin-dependent diabetes mellitus? Implications and recommendations for research. *J Pediatr Psychol.* 1999; **24**(3): 253–8.

Rovet JF, Ehrlich RM, Hoppe M. Intellectual deficits associated with early onset of insulin-dependent diabetes mellitus in children. *Diabetes Care.* 1987; **10**(4): 510–15.

Rubin RR, Peyrot M. Psychosocial problems and interventions in diabetes: a review of the literature. *Diabetes Care.* 1992; **15**: 1640–57.

Schlossberg NK. *Counseling Adults in Transition: linking practice with theory.* New York, NY: Springer; 1995.

Spierer H. *Major Transition in the Human Life Cycle.* New York, NY: Academic Press for Educational Development; 1977.

Vandagriff JL, Marrero DG, Ingersoll GM, *et al.* Parents of children with diabetes: what are they worried about? *Diabetes Educ.* 1992; **18**(4): 299–302.

Wolfsdorf JL, Anderson BA, Pasquarello C. Treatment of the child with diabetes. In: Kahn CR, Weir G, editors. *Joslin's Diabetes Mellitus.* 13th ed. Philadelphia, PA: Lea & Feiberg; 1994. pp. 430–51.

Wysocki T, Huxtable K, Linscheid TR, *et al.* Adjustment to diabetes mellitus in preschoolers and their mothers. *Diabetes Care.* 1989; **12**(8): 524–9.

CHAPTER 3

Challenges to emotional well-being: depression, anxiety and parental fear of hypoglycaemia

Carine De Beaufort and Katherine Barnard

INTRODUCTION

Children and young people suffering diabetes, their families and the health-care professionals they work with confront significant challenges. Living with the daily burden of managing diabetes inevitably takes its toll emotionally and psychologically on the whole family. Parents report increased health and psychological illnesses, greater anxiety, increased rates of depression and poorer quality of life than their counterparts (Barnard *et al.*, 2010). The capacity to overcome these challenges is influenced by many different factors, such as lifestyle, health beliefs, socio-economic situation, family structure and cohesion, age and peer group (Kilbourne *et al.*, 2009; Eckshtain *et al.*, 2010; Aman *et al.*, 2009; Cameron *et al.*, 2008; Hoey *et al.*, 2001).

Successful management of diabetes is also influenced by previous life experience (Goldston *et al.*, 1995). The development of intensive regimens has led to improved metabolic control (White *et al.*, 2001). However, while good metabolic control is positively associated with better quality of life, emotional well-being is at risk when confronted by the multitude of issues imposed by daily diabetes management (Hoey *et al.*, 2001). Furthermore, intensification of therapy can be negatively correlated with quality of life, not least because of the additional demands that intensification places on individuals and their families.

The way that healthcare professionals provide support and expertise to support families can help ensure positive outcomes, both medically and psychosocially. With careful self-management and appropriate medical support, families can minimise the impact of the many restrictions and limitations caused by type 1 diabetes. Healthcare professionals should be vigilant for the signs of possible emotional disturbances, such as depression or anxiety, which will require psychological assessment and treatment (Lernmark *et al.*, 1999; Pouwer *et al.*, 2006).

In this chapter, we will review the most common forms of emotional distress: depression and anxiety. We will look at their main identified symptoms and prevalence rates, as well as the diagnostic tools and the therapeutic approaches suggested by the literature. We will also cite diabetes-related emotional distress, and we will end with special attention to the fear of hypoglycaemia experienced by parents of children and young people with diabetes.

DEPRESSION

How to identify depression: signs and symptoms

Despite an increased awareness of depression and depressive symptoms, it may still be underestimated and under-diagnosed in children and young people, because of an atypical clinical presentation (Saluja *et al.*, 2004). Children and young people will experience a different combination of symptoms compared to adults, making it difficult to identify emotional distress (Ryan *et al.*, 1987). The signs and symptoms of depression in children and young people fall into four categories: (i) emotional signs; (ii) cognitive signs (those involving thinking); (iii) physical complaints; (iv) and behavioural changes (*see* Box 3.1).

BOX 3.1 Signs and symptoms of depression

Emotional signs
- May include sadness, withdrawal from friends, claims of feeling bored or disinterested in a previously enjoyable activity, complaints of feeling tense, panicky or reports of feeling worried and irritable.
- They may become broody or have a short temper and lash out in anger.

Cognitive signs
- Low mood can bring on negative, self-defeating thoughts, which can make it difficult to organise thoughts and may cause problems concentrating or remembering things in school.
- A negative view about self or others can result in feelings of worthlessness or guilt.

- Feeling helpless and/or hopeless and alone is common, as well as being sensitive to slights from peers. Some young people may talk about not wanting to be alive.

Physical signs
- Children may lose an interest in eating or, conversely, start eating too much.
- They may have difficulty falling asleep and staying asleep or they may wake too early or oversleep.
- They can also find it hard to stay awake during the day at school.
- They may talk and walk more slowly and they may be less active and playful than usual.
- In contrast, some children may be more fidgety or they may not be able to sit still.

Behavioural signs
- A common behavioural sign is avoiding everyday or enjoyable activities and responsibilities and withdrawing from friends and family.
- Depression can make a child or young person clingy and/or demanding.
- They may appear out of control in certain activities and spend long hours playing a video game or overeating.
- Restlessness may lead to fidgeting, acting up in class or reckless behaviour, including hurting themselves or taking excessive risks.

Environmental and family factors

Although pre-existing genetic risk factors may contribute to the development of depression, environmental factors such as family functioning alongside the potential burden of diabetes over time may exacerbate the development of depressive symptoms in children and young people with diabetes (Rice, 2010; Stewart et al., 2005). In addition, the parents of young children with type 1 diabetes experience depression and depressive symptomatology as a consequence of the additional caring burden associated with type 1 diabetes. In a recent systematic review of parental fear of hypoglycaemia, parents reported feelings of despair, isolation, fear and, in extreme cases, some had considered suicide, as the burden of caring for their child with diabetes had become too much to cope with (Barnard et al., 2010).

The diagnosis and treatment of depressive mood can have a major impact on metabolic outcome. The International Society for Pediatric and Adolescent Diabetes (ISPAD, 2000) clinical consensus guidelines stress that teams taking care of children and adolescents with diabetes should receive sufficient training to be able to recognise symptoms that may need attention and treatment

(Delamater, 2009). Untreated parental and, more specifically, maternal depression and depressive mood have been shown to have a major impact on metabolic and psychosocial outcome in the child or young person (Driscoll *et al.*, 2010; Butler *et al.*, 2009; Liakopoulou *et al.*, 2001).

Prevalence of depression

Estimates of the prevalence of depression in children and adolescents vary greatly, from 1% to 25% (Presicci *et al.*, 2010), and with an increased prevalence in girls post-puberty. There is an increase of up to five times higher than these prevalence figures in chronic disease and diabetes (Bennett, 1994). However, caution is required, as the differences in the published numbers vary depending on study methodology. Different measures used to screen for depression or depressive symptoms as well as atypical presentation in children has led to varying outcomes in reported prevalence. Kovacs and colleagues (1997) reported 47.5% psychiatric morbidity over a 10-year longitudinal survey, including depressive disorder, conduct and generalised anxiety disorders. In contrast, active screening, either by self-report in the clinic or by interview or web-based questionnaires, shows even further augmentation in prevalence (de Wit and Snoek, 2010). Without treatment, depressive symptoms interfere with the ability to effectively follow a safe diabetic regimen and ultimately they impact on metabolic control. Therefore, the need to consider carefully how to ensure regular screening in the diabetes clinic for low mood, depression and self-harming behaviours – including suicidality – has been strongly proposed (Cameron *et al.*, 2007; Goldston *et al.*, 1994; Radobuljac *et al.*, 2009).

Diabetes-related distress

Research has demonstrated that a substantial proportion of individuals do not report depressive symptoms, yet they still feel unable to cope with their diabetes. It has been suggested that these people are experiencing diabetes-related distress or are 'burned out' by their diabetes. *Diabetes burnout* occurs when a person feels 'overwhelmed by diabetes and by the frustrating burden of diabetes self-care' (Polonsky, 1995). This can be exacerbated by diabetes-specific family conflict, which is often associated with high levels of diabetes-related distress (Williams *et al.*, 2009). Though these emotions may be very different to feelings of depression, they can still be very destructive and they can have serious implications for care (Hilliard *et al.*, 2010).

Diagnostic tools

Over 20 years ago, representatives of government health departments and patients' organisations from all European countries met with diabetes experts at the International Diabetes Federation in St Vincent, Italy, in October 1989.

They unanimously agreed on several recommendations for diabetes care and urged for their implementation in all European countries. The St Vincent and Kos declaration argued that tools were needed to allow regular screening of emotional well-being and quality of life to facilitate improved care for all people with diabetes (Weber *et al.*, 1995).

Since this time, multidisciplinary diabetes teams have been developed in many hospitals and clinics. These work in partnership with families and are ideally placed to attend to changes in mood or behaviours in children and adolescents. Changes in metabolic control, an increase in cancelled appointments or failure to attend appointments may signal emerging emotional difficulties associated with problems living with diabetes. An increase in hospital admissions should trigger an assessment of potential psychological distress that may be connected with difficulty administering insulin or may be due to deliberate over- or under-administration (Stewart *et al.*, 2005).

Therapeutic approaches for depression

Cognitive behavioural therapy interventions, family therapy and pharmacological interventions have been shown to be effective in the treatment of depression (de Wit and Snoek, 2010; Manassis *et al.*, 2010). In a meta-analysis completed by Bridge *et al.* (2007), the efficacy of medication on suicidal ideation and/or suicide attempts in the general paediatric population with depressive disorders showed moderate beneficial effects dependent on age and chronicity. Early detection and intervention are both associated with better outcomes.

Rates of recurrence of depression in the diabetes population are described as being at the same level as those found in young people without diabetes. Therefore, a similar degree of long-term follow-up is recommended (Kovacs *et al.*, 1997). The interaction between depressive mood and metabolic outcome is well established, but there are few specific trials of psychological interventions specifically for young people diagnosed with diabetes and depression (Merry *et al.*, 2004) (*see* Chapters 11 and 12 to review the range of therapeutic approaches found to be helpful when working with young people with diabetes, low mood and poor metabolic control).

ANXIETY

Signs and symptoms of anxiety

Anxiety can be a normal reaction to stress, but sometimes it becomes a disabling disorder when it impacts excessively on a person's everyday living. Anxiety disorders are highly persistent, typically chronic and frequently coexist with one another and with other psychiatric conditions. However, they are significantly under-reported and under-diagnosed in children and young people

(Axelson and Birmaher, 2001). In addition, anxiety is often a precursor of or is co-morbid with depression (Williamson *et al.*, 2005).

Anxiety is experienced as a series of physical and emotional symptoms. Often it is normal to have these sensations on occasion, and so it is important to distinguish between normal and abnormal levels that affect day-to-day functioning. When considering anxiety in children and young people with diabetes, it is important to recognise that metabolic disturbances such as hypoglycaemia and fast-changing blood glucose measurements can simulate anxiety symptoms.

BOX 3.2 Signs and symptoms of anxiety in children and young people

Physical signs of anxiety
- Include headaches, sweating and feeling sick.
- Anxiety can raise the blood pressure and heart rate and can give you stomach pain, ulcers, diarrhoea, tingling in your fingers, weakness and shortness of breath.

Emotional signs of anxiety
- Feeling nervous, worried, apprehensive and scared or distressed.

Cognitive symptoms
- Anxiety can make it hard to think straight, to make decisions, to pay attention and concentrate, making it difficult to learn things in school.

Behavioural symptoms
- The most common behavioural manifestation of anxiety is withdrawal and/or avoidance of certain behaviours or activities (e.g. unable to leave the house or be in certain places). Alternatively, anxiety may also drive an increase in certain behaviours (e.g. checking, counting or hand-washing).

Prevalence of anxiety

Studies have reported on the prevalence of general anxiety as well as diabetes-specific symptoms, including fears, phobias, obsessions, possible symptoms interfering with treatment, or symptoms being caused by the diabetes and/or the treatment. Prevalence rates of 13.4%–19% have been described (Northam *et al.*, 2005; Goldston *et al.*, 1997). As with depression, there is a significant relationship between poor metabolic control and higher levels of worry and anxiety (Herzer and Hood, 2010; Hoey *et al.*, 2001).

Anxiety disorders

A diagnosis of abnormal anxiety requiring intervention depends on the child's age and developmental level, and (a) the impact of the anxiety on the level of daily functioning and (b) the amount of distress caused by the symptoms. 'Anxiety' is an umbrella term that encompasses a number of distinct anxiety disorders. They include the following.

Generalised anxiety disorder

The child or young person reports excessive worry and apprehension for a period of more than 6 months and has difficulty controlling the anxiety. They can appear restless or on edge, easily fatigued and have difficulty concentrating. They may be irritable, tense and have difficulty falling (or staying) asleep or they may have restless sleep.

Panic attacks

A sudden episode of intense fear and/or discomfort with an overwhelming desire to escape from impending danger that peaks over 10 minutes and then lasts about 20–30 minutes. The feeling of fear is accompanied by at least four physical or cognitive symptoms that may include increased heart rate, sweating, trembling or shaking, shortness of breath, a choking sensation, chest pain, nausea or stomach pain, dizziness or lightheadedness, faintness or unsteadiness, feelings of unreality, fear of going crazy, fear of dying, numbness or tingling sensations, chills or hot flashes.

Panic disorder

This consists of cycles of unexpected panic attacks with episodes of worry about having others. The thoughts and beliefs associated with the panic lead to changes in behaviour (e.g. anxiety and avoidance of situations from which escape may be difficult or help may not be available).

Obsessive–compulsive disorder

Persistent intrusive, unwanted thoughts, images, ideas or urges (obsessions) and/or intense uncontrollable repetitive behaviours or mental acts related to the obsessions (compulsions) that are unreasonable and excessive. The obsessions and compulsions cause distress, can have an impact on functioning and are time-consuming. The most common obsessions involve worry about contamination, doubts, arranging things in a specific order, fearful aggressive or murderous impulses, and disturbing sexual imagery (in older adolescents). Frequent compulsions include repetitive hand-washing or avoiding touching doors with hands, checking locks, windows and doors, engaging in counting rituals or repeating actions and requesting reassurance.

Post-traumatic stress disorder

This occurs after exposure to a traumatic event involving actual or perceived threat of death or serious bodily injury, where the response involves intense fear, helplessness or horror. The traumatic event is continually re-experienced so vividly that the individual may believe it is recurring. This causes him or her to experience distressing and intrusive recurrent images, thoughts, perceptions or dreams, and to experience intense emotional and physical anxiety and distress in situations that remind them of the event. Activities, places, thoughts or people associated with the event are avoided in an attempt to avert these experiences. The individual may struggle to remember details of the event and may lose interest in usual activities or feel detached from other people. They may have difficulty falling or staying asleep, be irritable, have difficulty concentrating or show excessive vigilance as well as having an exaggerated startle response. These symptoms persist for longer than a month after the event.

Acute stress disorder

This involves the same symptoms as post-traumatic stress disorder, persisting for less than 1 month.

Social phobia

If exposed to social situations with unfamiliar people, the individual feels they will do something that is embarrassing or humiliating. Exposure to the feared social situation may cause a panic attack. The belief may lead to avoidance of such situations or severe anxiety, leading to a marked interference in ability to function on a day-to-day basis.

Specific phobia

This is where exposure to the presence or potential presence of a specific feared situation or object provokes an acute anxiety reaction that is 'unreasonable and excessive'. The distress, determined avoidance and/or anxious anticipation of the event or object can significantly interfere with normal functioning or routine. Common phobias include injections, blood, hospital procedures, animals, insects, storms, heights, water, lifts, flying, bridges, escalators, trains, tunnels and enclosed spaces.

Adjustment disorder with anxiety (with or without depressed mood)

This is emotional and/or behavioural symptoms that occur within 3 months in response to an identifiable event or stressor that then go away once the stressor has gone.

Diabetes–specific anxiety

The diagnosis of a medical condition and its associated treatment regimen can also be identified as the cause of prominent anxiety symptoms. It is important to separate general childhood anxieties from diabetes-specific anxieties. The 'additional burden of diabetes' creates significant challenges for children, young people and their families. There are many general diabetes anxieties, such as wanting to maintain good control to avoid the threat of complications, or anxiety around injecting at school or how young people feel they are perceived by others and so forth.

Pre-existing generalised or specific anxiety disorders, disease-related anxiety and treatment-related anxiety have all been identified as having a negative impact on metabolic outcome and subsequent quality of life of children, young people and families (Horsch et al., 2007). Fear of needles and injections is also a common specific phobia, which is significantly exacerbated by a diagnosis of diabetes. Fear of needles can result in high levels of avoidance behaviour and a refusal to have insulin injections or complete blood tests (Hanas and Ludvigsson, 1997; Hanas et al., 2011). The anxiety is often extreme and easily observed, especially in younger children, where there is loud and obvious protest. In older children and adolescents, anxiety about needles may only become apparent through increasingly poor metabolic control, high blood glucose measurements or a failure to regularly monitor blood glucose.

Diagnostic tools

While there are some screening measures that can be used to assess possible generalised and diabetes-specific anxiety disorders in a clinic setting, further research is needed to identify optimal tools for the assessment of worry and anxiety. These should be used alongside more consistent methodological approaches to allow a more accurate estimate of the prevalence of both generalised and diabetes-specific anxiety in clinical populations (a review of screening measures can be found in Part III of this book).

Regular use of brief, self-reported, diabetes-specific measures alongside clinical assessment should enable early identification and treatment of anxiety disorders in children, young people and their parents. Untreated anxiety disorders are likely to become entrenched and have a negative lifelong impact on diabetes management and outcome.

Therapeutic approaches

The majority of therapeutic approaches for anxiety disorders are individually based. The focus of evidence-based treatment approaches is on identifying the negative thoughts that are driving the overwhelming emotional distress and triggering avoidance behaviours designed to reduce the worry. However, as with depression, there are no specific interventions designed for generalised anxiety in children with diabetes. Some treatment approaches for diabetes-specific anxieties have been developed. Targeting specific behaviours through educational workshops using behaviour therapy techniques has been shown to reduce anxiety-induced symptoms in paediatric diabetes patients (Wysocki, 2006).

For young people struggling with fear of needles or injections, practical changes can help (*see* Chapter 1). When these changes do not improve the situation, distraction techniques and behavioural management can help; however, if the child or young person does not respond to this well-documented approach for needle phobias, more intensive therapeutic interventions may be needed (*see* Chapter 12). At the current time, there are no evidence-based interventions to help manage fear of hypoglycaemia.

ANXIETY, DEPRESSION AND FEARS IN FAMILIES

Parental anxiety and depression

Increased maternal depression and anxiety are associated with greater fear of hypoglycaemia (Jaser *et al.*, 2009), with maternal symptoms of anxiety and depression unrelated to their child's metabolic control. '*Not being there*' if the child needs them is a major cause of anxiety for many parents, as well as them having hypoglycaemia during the night and consequently not waking up in the morning. Negative associations exist between families' socio-economic status and the extent to which they worry about hypoglycaemia (Patton *et al.*, 2007). Family income and education play a role too, with families on lower income levels finding it more upsetting to cope with diabetes-related stress and experiencing higher levels of anxiety and stress, particularly in mothers (Jaser *et al.*, 2009). Conversely, it has been reported that parents with children who maintained HbA$_{1c}$ within a target range had higher incomes and knowledge levels than those with children with HbA$_{1c}$ levels outside the target range (Stallwood, 2006).

Fear of hypoglycaemia

Parents have a number of diabetes-specific worries and anxieties that include anxiety associated with frequent blood glucose monitoring: the cited fear of '*not being there*' despite daily management being relentless and fear that others, such as babysitters or teachers, will be unable to provide appropriate care for their child. Experiencing hypoglycaemia at some point in time after diagnosis and engaging in subsequent avoidance behaviours contributes to fear of hypoglycaemia. Some parents report that they will run blood glucose levels 'slightly' higher than recommended to avoid acute episodes of hypoglycaemia and associated seizures both during the day and at night (Barnard *et al.*, 2010; Irvine *et al.*, 1992).

The knock-on effect of this will be a higher HbA_{1c}. Paradoxically, chronically higher HbA_{1c} levels are associated with the signs of acute hypoglycaemia presenting at higher blood glucose levels – that is, rather than 3.9 and below. This means hypoglycaemic signs can be present when the patient is actually hyperglycaemic rather than hypoglycaemic. Thus, parents engage in further avoidance behaviours, leading to even higher HbA_{1c}, causing a spiral effect of worsening diabetes control. With every 1% increase in HbA_{1c}, there is an associated 60% increase in risk of long-term complications. This behaviour can be either conscious or subconscious, with fear a strong motivating factor to maintain such maladaptive coping despite the long-term risks.

A recent literature review of the contributing factors to parental fear described that mothers of young children with type 1 diabetes reported greater fear of hypoglycaemia and took more steps to avoid it than fathers did (Patton et al., 2008). However, although mothers and fathers reported the same level of worry about hypoglycaemia, fathers experienced greater levels of parenting stress and had lower confidence in their ability to manage their child's diabetes, reporting greater anxiety and increased hopelessness than mothers.

Half of the parents reported the child experiencing an episode of hypoglycaemia three to four times per week (Patton et al., 2007). However, the severity of hypoglycaemia seemed more important in causing fear than its frequency, especially in parents whose child had experienced a hypoglycaemic seizure. Almost a third of children with diabetes (32%) had experienced at least one hypoglycaemia seizure during their lifetime (Patton et al., 2008). It is perhaps unsurprising that parents of children who had experienced a hypoglycaemic seizure within the past year had significantly greater overall fear of hypoglycaemia (both in terms of avoidance behaviour and in terms of the extent to which they worry about it) than those whose children had not experienced a seizure. Mothers whose children had a history of passing out experienced far greater worry than mothers whose children had never lost consciousness. Furthermore, children who had experienced a seizure with loss of consciousness had a significantly higher rate of self-monitoring of blood glucose values above the desired target range than young children with no history of seizures, which suggests that parents of these children are indeed allowing higher-than-desired blood glucose levels to avoid hypoglycaemia.

The degree of distress experienced by mothers about hypoglycaemia occurring while their child was asleep or in social situations has been found to be related to the mother's level of fear but not to maternal confidence in ability to treat hypoglycaemia or to confidence in being able to recognise hypos (Monoghan et al., 2009). The most common fear reported by parents relating to hypoglycaemia was feeling the child will have a low blood glucose while asleep or when away from a parent (reported by 46% of parents in Patton et al.,

2007). Cultural, ethnic and socio-economic differences exist, with Caucasian parents and those with higher education reporting greater levels of fear associated with hypoglycaemia. Fewer years of education and lower income were reported to produce greater (i.e. background level) anxiety.

Common strategies to prevent hypoglycaemia

Common strategies used by parents to prevent hypoglycaemia include carrying fast-acting sugar, checking blood glucose often when attending a long event, avoiding being away from their child when his/her blood glucose might go low and feeding the child at the first sign of hypoglycaemia (Patton *et al.*, 2007). Monaghan *et al.* (2009) reported that parents often engage in nocturnal blood glucose monitoring, and those who reported 'often/always' were more likely to have a child on a basal-bolus regimen and it was more likely for their child to have a significantly longer illness duration.

SUMMARY

Living with diabetes brings a significant medical and psychosocial burden. The presence of higher levels of depression and anxiety in children and young people diagnosed with diabetes is well documented, as it is for their parents also. Low mood, general and diabetes-specific anxieties have a significant impact on quality of life, perceived well-being and long-term metabolic control.

Parents of children with type 1 diabetes report a high level of anxiety and fear associated with managing the condition. It is common for them to engage in avoidance behaviours that result in their child's blood glucose control being persistently higher than recommended, leading to subsequent risks for the development of diabetes-related complications.

Early identification of emotional difficulties and diabetes-related distress is essential, as is the development and provision of effective, evidence-based therapeutic interventions that can be provided as part of integrated diabetes healthcare delivery.

REFERENCES

Aman J, Skinner TC, de Beaufort CE, *et al.* Associations between physical activity, sedentary behavior, and glycemic control in a large cohort of adolescents with type 1 diabetes: the Hvidoere Study Group on Childhood Diabetes. *Pediatr Diabetes.* 2009; **10**(4): 234–9.

Axelson DA, Birmaher B. Relation between anxiety and depressive disorders in childhood and adolescence. *Depress Anxiety.* 2001; **14**(2): 67–78.

Barnard K, Thomas S, Royle P, *et al.* Fear of hypoglycaemia in parents of young children with type 1 diabetes: a systematic review. *BMC Pediatr.* 2010; **10**: 50–60.

Bennett DS. (1994) Depression among children with chronic medical problems: a meta-analysis. *J Pediatr Psychol.* **19**: 149–69.

Bridge JA, Iyengar S, Salary CB, *et al.* Clinical response and risk for reported suicidal ideation and suicide attempts in pediatric antidepressant treatment: a meta-analysis of randomized controlled trials. *JAMA.* 2007; **297**(15): 1683–96.

Butler JM, Berg CA, King P, *et al.* Parental negative affect and adolescent efficacy for diabetes management. *J Fam Psychol.* 2009; **23**(4): 611–14.

Cameron FJ, Northam EA, Ambler GR, *et al.* Routine psychological screening in youth with type 1 diabetes and their parents: a notion whose time has come? *Diabetes Care.* 2007; **30**(10): 2716–24.

Cameron FJ, Skinner TC, de Beaufort CE, *et al.* Hvidoere Study Group on childhood diabetes: are family factors universally related to metabolic outcomes in adolescents with type 1 diabetes? *Diabet Med.* 2008; **25**(4): 463–8.

De Wit M, Snoek FJ. Depressive symptoms and unmet psychological needs of Dutch youth with type 1 diabetes: results of a web-survey. *Pediatr Diabetes.* Epub 2010 Jun.

Delamater AM. Psychological care of children and adolescents with diabetes. *Pediatr Diabetes.* 2009; **10**(Suppl. 12): 175–84.

Driscoll KA, Johnson SB, Barker D, *et al.* Risk factors associated with depressive symptoms in caregivers of children with type 1 diabetes or cystic fibrosis. *J Pediatr Psychol.* Epub 2010 Jan 22.

Eckshtain D, Ellis DA, Kolmodin K, *et al.* The effects of parental depression and parenting practices on depressive symptoms and metabolic control in urban youth with insulin dependent diabetes. *J Pediatr Psychol.* 2010; **35**(4): 426–35.

Goldston DB, Kelley AU, Rebouisson DM, *et al.* Suicidal ideation and behaviour and non compliance with the medical regimen among diabetic adolescents. *J Am Acad Child Adolesc Psychiatry.* 1997; **36**(11): 1528–36.

Goldston DB, Kovacs M, Ho VY, *et al.* Suicidal ideation and suicide attempts among youth with insulin dependent diabetes. *J Am Acad Child Adolesc Psychiatry.* 1994; **33**(2): 240–6.

Goldston DB, Kovacs M, Obrosky DS, *et al.* A longitudinal study of life events and metabolic control among youths with insulin-dependent diabetes mellitus. *Health Psychol.* 1995; **14**(5): 409–14.

Hanas R, de Beaufort C, Hoey H, *et al.* Insulin delivery by injection in children and adolescents with diabetes. *Pediatr Diabetes.* 2011; **10**: 1111–399.

Hanas R, Ludvigsson J. Experience of pain from insulin injection and needle phobia in young patients with IDDM. *Pract Diab Int.* 1997; **14**: 95–9.

Herzer M, Hood K. Anxiety symptoms in adolescents with type 1 diabetes: association with blood glucose monitoring and glycemic control. *J Pediatr Psychol.* 2010; **35**(4): 415–25.

Hilliard ME, Monaghan M, Cogen FR, *et al.* Parent stress and child behaviour among young children with type 1 diabetes. *Child Care Health Dev.* Epub 2010 Nov 18.

Hoey H, Aanstoot HJ, Chiarelli F, *et al.* Good metabolic control is associated with better quality of life in 2,101 adolescents with type 1 diabetes. *Diabetes Care.* 2001; **24**(11): 1923–8.

Horsch A, Mcmanus F, Kennedy P, *et al.* Anxiety, depressive, and posttraumatic stress symptoms in mothers of children with type 1 diabetes. *J Trauma Stress.* 2007; **20**(5): 881–91.

International Society for Pediatric and Adolescent Diabetes (ISPAD). *Consensus Guidelines for the Management of Type 1 Diabetes Mellitus in Children and Adolescents.* Berlin: ISPAD; 2011.

Available at: www.ispad.org/NewsFiles/IDF-ISPAD_Diabetes_in_Childhood_and%20 Adolescence_Guidelines_2011.pdf

Irvine AA, Cox DJ, Gonder-Frederick L. Fear of hypoglycemia: relationship to physical and psychological symptoms in patients with insulin dependent diabetes mellitus. *Health Psychol.* 1992; **11**(2): 135–8.

Jaser SS, Whittemore R, Ambrosino JM, *et al.* Coping and psychosocial adjustment in mothers of young children with type 1 diabetes. *Child Health Care.* 2009; **38**(2): 91–106.

Kilbourne B, Cummings SM, Levine RS. The influence of religiosity on depression among low-income people with diabetes. *Health Soc Work.* 2009; **34**(2): 137–47.

Kovacs M, Goldston D, Obrosky DS, *et al.* Psychiatric disorders in youths with IDDM: rates and risk factors. *Diabetes Care.* 1997; **20**(1): 36–44.

Lernmark B, Persson BM, Fishert L, *et al.* Symptoms of depression are important to psychological adaptation and metabolic control in children with diabetes mellitus. *Diabet Med.* 1999; **16**(1): 14–22.

Liakopoulou M, Alifieraki Z, Katideniou A, *et al.* Maternal expressed emotion and metabolic control of children and adolescents with diabetes mellitus. *Psychother Psychosom.* 2001; **70**(2): 78–85.

Manassis K, Wilansky-Traynor P, Farzan N, *et al.* The feelings club randomized controlled evaluation of schoolbased CBT for anxious or depressive symptoms. *Depress Anxiety.* 2010; **27**(10): 945–52.

Merry S, McDowell H, Hetrick S, *et al.* Psychological and/or educational interventions for the prevention of depression in children and adolescents. *Cochrane Database Syst Rev.* 2004; (1): CD003380.

Monaghan MC, Hilliard ME, Cogen FR, *et al.* Nighttime caregiving behaviors among parents of young children with type 1 diabetes: associations with illness characteristics and parent functioning. *Fam Syst Health.* 2009; **27**(1): 28–38.

Northam EA, Matthews LK, Anderson PJ, *et al.* Psychiatric morbidity and health outcome in type 1 diabetes: perspectives from a prospective longitudinal study. *Diabet Med.* 2005; **22**(2): 152–7.

Patton SR, Dolan LM, Henry R, *et al.* Parental fear of hypoglycemia: young children treated with continuous subcutaneous insulin infusion. *Pediatr Diabetes.* 2007; **8**(6): 362–8.

Patton SR, Dolan LM, Henry R, *et al.* Fear of hypoglycemia in parents of young children with type 1 diabetes mellitus. *J Clin Psychol Med Settings.* 2008; **15**(3): 252–9.

Polonsky W, Anderson B, Lohrer P, *et al.* Assessment of diabetes-related distress. *Diabetes Care.* 1995; **18**(6): 754–60.

Pouwer F, Beekman AT, Lubach C. *et al.* Nurses' recognition and registration of depression anxiety and diabetes specific problems in outpatients with diabetes mellitus. *Patient Educ Couns.* 2006; **60**(2): 235–40.

Presicci A, Lecce P, Ventura P, *et al.* Depressive and adjustment disorder: some questions about the differential diagnosis: case studies. *Neuropsychiatr Dis Treat.* 2010; **6**: 473–81.

Radobuljac MD, Bratina NU, Battelino T, *et al.* Lifetime prevalence of suicidal and self-injurious behaviors in a representative cohort of Slovenian adolescents with type 1 diabetes. *Pediatr Diabetes.* 2009; **10**(7): 424–31.

Rice F. Genetics of childhood and adolescent depression: insights into etiological heterogeneity and challenges for future genomic research. *Genome Med.* 2010; **2**(9): 68.

Ryan ND, Puig-Antich J, Ambrosini P, *et al.* The clinical picture of major depression in children and adolescents. *Arch Gen Psychiatry.* 1987; **44**(10): 854–61.

Saluja G, Iachan R, Scheidt PC, *et al.* Prevalence of and risk factors for depressive symptoms among young adolescents. *Arch Pediatr Adolesc Med.* 2004; **158**(8): 760–5.

Stallwood L. Relationship between caregiver knowledge and socioeconomic factors on glycemic outcomes of young children with diabetes. *J Spec Pediatr Nurs.* 2006; **11**(3): 158–65.

Stewart SM, Rao U, White P. Depression and diabetes in children and adolescents. *Curr Opin Pediatr.* 2005; **17**(5): 626–31.

Stewart SM, Rao U, Emslie GJ, *et al.* Depressive symptoms predict hospitalization for adolescents with type 1 diabetes mellitus. *Pediatrics.* 2005; **115**(5): 1315–19.

Weber B, Brink S, Bartsocas C, *et al.* ISPAD declaration of Kos. *J Paediatr Child Health.* 1995; **31**(2): 156.

White NH, Cleary PA, Dahms W, *et al.* Beneficial effects of intensive therapy of diabetes during adolescence: outcomes after the conclusion of the Diabetes Control and Complications Trial (DCCT). *J Pediatr.* 2001; **139**(6): 804–12.

Williamson DE, Forbes EE, Dahl RE, *et al.* A genetic epidemiological perspective on comorbidity of depression and anxiety. *Child Adolesc Psychiatr Clin North Am.* 2005; **14**(4): 707–26.

Williams LB, Laffel LM, Hood KK. Diabetes-specific family conflict and psychological distress in paediatric type 1 diabetes. *Diabet Med.* 2009; **26**(9): 908–14.

Wysocki T. Behavioral assessment and intervention in pediatric diabetes. *Behav Modif.* 2006; **30**(1): 72–92.

CHAPTER 4

Regimen adherence: paradigms and approaches

Alan Delamater, Anna Maria Patino-Fernandez, Elizabeth Pulgaron and Amber Daigre

INTRODUCTION

The regimen for managing diabetes is complex and consists of multiple components that have been described in detail in Chapter 1. The ultimate aim of balancing all of the components of a complex diabetes regimen should be to achieve blood glucose levels as near to normal as possible while at the same time avoiding extreme variability of hypo- and hyperglycaemia. Different perspectives on the challenging nature of this task will be presented throughout this book. Achieving normal glycaemic control requires the integration of considerable amounts of information concerning factors affecting blood glucose levels and then applying problem-solving techniques to achieve glycaemic goals. This is particularly challenging for young people and for children where parental involvement is one of the key elements to successful diabetes management.

Not surprisingly, research has indicated that optimal regimen adherence is difficult to achieve for many young people with diabetes. For example, early studies showed that dietary skills deficits and adherence problems were common (Delamater *et al.*, 1988; Schmidt *et al.*, 1992). Blood glucose monitoring was typically not performed as often as prescribed, and blood glucose data were not routinely used to make appropriate changes in the regimen (Delamater *et al.*, 1989). Insulin is often omitted, particularly for adolescent girls who are concerned with body weight issues (Bryden *et al.*, 1999; Neumark-Szatainer *et al.*, 2002; Weissberg-Benchell *et al.*, 1995).

This chapter addresses regimen adherence in children and adolescents with type 1 diabetes. We begin by reviewing the concept of regimen adherence, with consideration of the related term 'compliance', and distinguish these from self-care behaviours. We then review various approaches to the assessment of regimen adherence, before going on to consider factors related to adherence, including demographic, psychosocial and healthcare system variables.

THE CONSTRUCT OF REGIMEN ADHERENCE

Three terms are used to describe what people do in relation to their prescribed medical regimen: 'compliance', 'adherence' and 'self-care behaviours'. Although they are often used interchangeably, it is important to distinguish among them, as they are conceptually different.

Compliance

The term compliance comes from the medical model and typically refers to the 'extent to which a person's behaviour . . . coincides with medical advice' (Haynes *et al.*, 1979, pp. 2–3). Compliance is a distinct class of behaviour in a child's entire repertoire of adherent behaviours.

Within a medical context, compliance can be categorised as:
1. compliance with requests to do something (e.g. to take medication, to wear an identification bracelet, to follow dietary recommendations)
2. compliance with a request to refrain from doing something (e.g. to limit sedentary activity).

Non-compliance is thus conceptualised as disobeying advice, and it implies a negative attitude towards the 'patient'. Usually a failure to comply is seen as the fault of the individual. The concept here is that he or she has a passive role in their relationship with the healthcare professional.

Non-compliance can be categorised as:
1. failure to initiate behaviour
2. failure to sustain compliance until the command has been fulfilled
3. failure to follow previously taught rules.

Most healthcare providers use the term 'compliance' and attribute non-compliance to personal qualities of the individual, such as forgetfulness, lack of willpower or discipline, or low level of education (Delamater *et al.*, 2001). There are several disadvantages to thinking in terms of compliance and non-compliance, including poor rapport with children, young people and their families and promoting resistance on the part of the young person and/or parent.

Adherence

'Adherence' is a term that implies the active, voluntary and collaborative involvement of the individual in producing therapeutic results (Meichenbaum and Turk, 1987). This term de-emphasises 'obedience' and highlights the active role of all family members in working with the medical team. From this perspective, the child, young person and family are empowered to feel a sense of mastery and to adhere to the regimen because it is for their well-being, and not because they are being told to do so, assuming an internalisation of the treatment recommendations. This also turns the focus on behaviour and takes away the blame from the young person when they are non-adherent. It allows the healthcare professional to target certain behaviours that they see as necessary for adherence. Rather than viewing adherence as a unitary construct, it is important to consider the multiple behaviours involved in the diabetes treatment regimen.

Self-care behaviour

Young children rely on parents to carry out the numerous self-care activities or behaviours associated with the diabetes regimen. As children mature and develop, these responsibilities are typically transferred to the adolescent. In general, research has shown that the diabetes regimen is multidimensional and adherence to one regimen component may be unrelated to adherence in other areas (Kurtz, 1990).

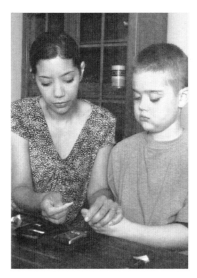

A mother tests her son's glucose levels

With the results of the Diabetes Control and Complications Trial concluding that maintenance of normal HbA_{1c} levels by intensive insulin therapy delays the onset and slows the progression of retinopathy, neuropathy and nephropathy (DCCT, 1994), 'tight' control of blood glucose has become the main goal of medical management of diabetes, with prevention of hypo- and hyperglycaemia. Intensive regimens (i.e. multiple injections and continuous blood glucose measures) are being prescribed in the hope of preventing or delaying the health complications of diabetes (*see* Chapter 8).

From a measurement point of view, it is important to distinguish self-care behaviours from the constructs of 'compliance' and 'adherence'. The latter terms are essentially relative, while the former can be considered absolute. In other words, adherence is relative to some ideal (i.e. the prescription) and could be considered as a proportional or percentage outcome. For example, if a patient is prescribed four blood glucose checks per day and does only two of them, this would indicate 50% adherence; however, if they were prescribed two blood glucose checks and performed two, this would indicate 100% adherence. On the other hand, measurement of self-care behaviours may assume an absolute approach in which the only concern would be the number of behaviours (e.g. blood glucose checks) performed in a given time period; two versus four blood glucose checks per day may have different implications, and empirically may show different relationships with measures of health outcomes such as HbA$_{1c}$.

ASSESSMENT OF REGIMEN ADHERENCE
Approaches to measurement of adherence
Across paediatric chronic illness, investigators are challenged with the difficult task of how best to measure regimen adherence. There are several approaches to the measurement of medical regimen adherence, ranging from direct to indirect methodologies:

- direct observation of behaviours
- 24-hour recall interviews
- structured interview
- patient self-report
- parent/caregiver report
- healthcare provider ratings
- treatment outcome.

Caregiver and self-report methods are the most common methods of assessing regimen adherence (Quittner *et al.*, 2007); they typically include such approaches as 24-hour recall interviews, retrospective paper-and-pencil questionnaires, electronic measures (e.g. insulin pump data, accelerometer to measure physical activity) or use of permanent products such as logbooks (written or electronic). Many researchers favour caregiver and self-report measures since they are inexpensive and can be administered to multiple informants. Structured interviews, another means of gathering caregiver and self-report information, provide flexibility since interviewers can ask follow-up questions. However, although they are popular, one must also consider the weaknesses of caregiver and self-report measures. Respondents tend to overestimate adherence, and reliance on recall often results in inaccurate reporting. Additionally, questionnaires and interviews may be difficult to administer to young children (Quittner *et al.*, 2007).

Similar to the questionnaire method used with children, young people and parents, several studies have utilised healthcare provider ratings as a measure of regimen adherence (Jacobson *et al.*, 1990; Hauser *et al.*, 1990). Though some investigators find them to be an improvement over parent and patient reports, they are often based on information provided by family members, and therefore may still reflect the same biases inherent in self-reporting. Furthermore, ratings from the clinical team may be influenced by prior non-adherence or treatment outcome (La Greca *et al.*, 2009).

Twenty-four-hour recall interviews seek to solve the issue of inaccurate retrospective reporting by shortening the recall period to only 1 day. Children and/ or parents are asked to describe the previous day, beginning with waking up and ending with bedtime. This approach shows good agreement with observed regimen adherence behaviours, with the exception of dietary behaviours, which are typically underestimated (i.e. underestimation of number and amount of meals and snacks consumed) (Reynolds *et al.*, 1990).

Daily diary methods can include several methodologies, including written or electronic logs, as well as telephone diaries completed with the respondent. Though this method minimises the recall period, previous studies indicate poor adherence with written logs, which are often completed all at one time just before returning to the researcher, rather than on a daily basis (Johnson *et al.*, 1992).

Much like 24-hour recall interviews, telephone and electronic logs seek to solve the problem of poor adherence associated with written diary methods. Telephone and electronic methods collect data in real time, allowing for no lapse in completion and decreasing the likelihood of memory decay. Furthermore, by eliminating the person-to-person interview, electronic methods decrease the likelihood of participants responding in a socially desirable fashion (Quittner *et al.*, 2007). Blood glucose meters and insulin pumps provide additional options for electronic monitoring of adherence because of their memory capabilities. To assess physical activity, it is possible to use accelerometers to monitor adherence to physical activity recommendations. This is difficult to do in regular clinical practice, and therefore pedometers may provide a more feasible alternative. Data can be downloaded to a computer from these machines to assess adherence to blood glucose monitoring, basal and bolus administrations or even physical activity levels over time.

Direct observation of regimen adherence yields accurate information about the child or young person's skills in the clinic setting; however, the information may not be generalised to the natural environment. To address this short-coming, researchers would have to observe people directly in their natural environments – a solution that is far too impractical and expensive and there-fore one that has been rarely used in clinical research (Reynolds *et al.*, 1990).

The various approaches to the measurement of regimen adherence in pae-diatric diabetes are described in detail in Part III of this book (practical tools).

FACTORS RELATED TO REGIMEN ADHERENCE

Various studies have revealed several factors related to regimen adherence. These factors can be categorised into three groups: (i) demographic; (ii) psy-chosocial; and (iii) healthcare system variables. Understanding these factors is important in order to develop effective prevention and intervention pro-grammes to improve patient adherence.

Demographic variables

Children and adolescents from ethnic minority backgrounds, with low socio-economic status and from single-parent families have been found to have poorer regimen adherence (Jacobson *et al.*, 1997). Age or developmental status is one of the strongest predictors of adherence, with children showing increased adherence problems as they get older. Adolescence in general is a particularly difficult time for young people to carry out self-care behaviours, for a number of reasons. Multiple factors contribute to age-related differences, such as age shifts in a child's responsibility for disease management, increasing pressures from peers to be accepted and biological changes associated with development (La Greca and Mackey, 2009). Biologically, hormonal changes associated with puberty result in decreased insulin sensitivity, thus negatively affecting blood glucose metabolism and leading to increased blood glucose levels (Amiel *et al.*, 1986).

Psychosocial variables

Cognitive processes such as learned helplessness,[1] self-efficacy,[2] health beliefs and risk perception have been found to be related to adherence. Appropriate health beliefs, such as perceived seriousness of diabetes, vulnerability to complications and the efficacy of treatment, have been found to predict better adherence (Brownlee-Duffeck *et al.*, 1987). Bond *et al.* (1992) found that the best adherence was observed when perceived threat was low and perceived benefits to costs were high. Cognitive appraisals such as the perception of little internal control over health and an external attribution style for negative events have also been associated with lower levels of regimen adherence (Murphy *et al.*, 1997). Self-esteem – the degree to which a child or young person feels good about themselves, feels confident, accepted and valued – has also been found to be important in adherence, with higher levels of adherence being reported in children who have better self-esteem (Littlefield, 1992).

Social development influences adherence, and there have been several studies examining the influence of friends on diabetes management. Pressure to conform to peers in specific social situations and to be accepted by peers is related to decreases in adherence during the adolescent years (Helgeson *et al.*, 2007; Thomas *et al.*, 1997). Social demand has also been shown to influence reports of adherence to glucose monitoring (Delamater *et al.*, 1998). Furthermore, when young people attribute negative peer reactions to their self-care, they are more likely to have adherence difficulties (Hains *et al.*, 2007; La Greca *et al.*, 2002). Peer support, in contrast, is positively related to adherence, but varies depending on the self-care behaviour in question. For example, social support has been found to be associated with greater adherence for dietary and exercise behaviours (La Greca *et al.*, 2002).

Coping skills are related to adherence, with greater adherence in children who have more adaptive coping skills and lower levels of maladaptive coping. In particular, a child's ability to cope with stress, such as that experienced with a new diagnosis, or negative life events (including daily hassles) is related to adherence. For example, research has shown that good coping and adjustment of children in the months just after diagnosis were predictive of better regimen adherence over the first 4 years of having diabetes (Jacobson *et al.*, 1990), and maladaptive coping has also been associated with poor regimen adherence (Hanson *et al.*, 1989).

Studies have shown that family functioning with low levels of family conflict (Lewandoski and Drotar, 2007), good communication patterns (Miller-Johnson *et al.*, 1994) and problem-solving (Wysocki *et al.*, 2008) among

---

1 A state of mind that results from repeated experiences of being unable to do anything to change one's circumstances.

2 A sense of mastery over events or circumstances.

family members is associated with better regimen adherence. Healthier family functioning in the months just after diagnosis was predictive of better regimen adherence over the first 4 years of having diabetes (Hauser *et al.*, 1990). In contrast, family conflict has been associated with lower adherence (Miller-Johnson *et al.*, 1994). Higher levels of adherence have been associated with greater family support for diabetes care in studies with adolescents (Ellis *et al.*, 2007; Skinner *et al.*, 2000).

Clear disease management responsibility and communication around expectations is critical for proper adherence. Parents, young people and the healthcare team should understand who assumes responsibility for the various management tasks and how that responsibility is shared within the family. Studies have shown that greater family involvement and shared responsibility (Helgeson *et al.*, 2008), including parental monitoring (Ellis *et al.*, 2007), are associated with better adherence. When children are given self-care autonomy without sufficient cognitive and social maturity, problems with regimen adherence are more likely (Wysocki *et al.*, 1996).

Psychopathology has also been studied in relation to regimen adherence, with major psychiatric disorders such as depression linked with poor regimen adherence (Kovacks *et al.*, 1992). Research has also shown that in adolescents with diabetes, the relationship between depression and glycaemic control is mediated by regimen adherence (McGrady *et al.*, 2009).

INTERVENTIONS TO IMPROVE ADHERENCE

Research findings indicate that various types of interventions have improved regimen adherence of young people with diabetes. Interventions focusing on increasing motivation through individual counselling or with the aid of technology or interacting with others through the Internet can improve adherence and diabetes outcomes. Family-based behavioural procedures, such as goal-setting, self-monitoring, positive reinforcement, behavioural contracts, supportive parental communications and appropriately shared responsibility for diabetes management, have improved regimen adherence and glycaemic control, as well as the parent–adolescent relationship. Research has also shown that interventions focusing on improving peer-group support, problem-solving and coping skills have improved diabetes management. These approaches are described in detail in Chapter 12.

Healthcare system variables

Various organisational factors play a role in a child's ability to adhere to a complex medical regimen. These include a family's proximity to the clinic, transport, scheduling of appointments and integration of care, as well as reminder postcards, phone calls about upcoming patient appointments and appointments that begin on time (Haynes *et al.*, 1979). Additionally, both the support received from the healthcare team and the patient–doctor relationship have been shown to be important factors related to regimen adherence (Kyngäs, 2007; Delamater, 2006). Specifically, parents and adolescents who are satisfied with the medical care they have received are more likely to adhere to the physician's recommendations (Naar-King *et al.*, 2006).

SUMMARY

Research findings indicate that regimen adherence problems are common among children and adolescents with type 1 diabetes. It is well known that adherence problems are more likely when regimens are complex and chronic, and this is certainly the case with diabetes. In particular, there are considerable problems with inadequate blood glucose monitoring, insulin omission and dietary skills, especially with older children and adolescents. Regimen adherence problems are often related to various psychosocial difficulties, including family conflict, lack of parental involvement and support of self-care behaviours, and behavioural or emotional problems, including depression and eating disorders. These may interact with such cognitive factors as health beliefs and perceived coping capacity. When parents or healthcare teams encourage adolescents to have self-care autonomy without sufficient cognitive and social maturity, they are likely to have more problems with diabetes management. Besides these psychosocial and cognitive factors, research has also demonstrated that adherence is related to demographic factors such as age and to healthcare system factors such as the patient–physician relationship.

Understanding the nature of adherence problems is important to facilitate optimal adherence. The terms 'compliance' and 'adherence' are often used interchangeably, but they are very different conceptually. Another way to view this situation is to consider self-care behaviours on a more absolute level than the relative level that compliance and adherence assume. This has important implications for how to work with people to improve diabetes management, as well as how to measure adherence or self-care behaviours.

There are a number of ways to reliably and validly measure regimen adherence, including questionnaires and interviews administered to people and parents, as well as using objective measures such as blood glucose meters to determine the number of tests performed over a defined period of time. Most of these measures have clinical utility as well, so they can be used routinely in clinical settings. Clinician ratings are generally not good estimates of regimen adherence, since they may be biased by knowledge of glycaemic control as well as personal history.

In conclusion, a substantial behavioural science research base has demonstrated that psychosocial factors play an integral role in the management of diabetes in children. Research has shown that there are a number of reliable and valid ways to measure regimen adherence in the clinical setting. Research has also shown the efficacy of a number of psychosocial therapies that can improve adherence and glycaemic control in children and adolescents with diabetes. More research is needed to develop interventions to improve diabetes management in specific patient populations and to demonstrate the cost-effectiveness of these approaches. More work is also needed to identify effective models to integrate psychosocial services into routine diabetes care.

REFERENCES

Amiel SA, Sherwin R, Simonson DC, *et al.* Impaired insulin action in puberty: a contributing factor to poor glycemic control in adolescents with diabetes. *New Engl J Med.* 1986; **315**(4): 215–19.

Bond G, Aiken L, Somerville S. The health belief model and adolescents with insulin-dependent diabetes mellitus. *Health Psychol.* 1992; **11**(3): 190–8.

Brownlee-Duffeck M, Peterson L, Simonds JF, *et al.* The role of health beliefs in the regimen adherence and metabolic control of adolescents and adults with diabetes mellitus. *J Consult Clin Psychol.* 1987; **55**(2): 139–44.

Bryden KS, Neil A, Mayou RA, *et al.* Eating habits, body weight, and insulin misuse: a longitudinal study of teenagers and young adults with type 1 diabetes. *Diabetes Care.* 1999; **22**(12): 1956–60.

Delamater A. Improving patient adherence. *Clin Diabetes.* 2006; **24**(2): 71–7.

Delamater AM, Davis SG, Bubb J, *et al.* Self-monitoring of blood glucose by adolescents with diabetes: technical skills and utilization of data. *Diabetes Educ.* 1989; **15**(1): 56–61.

Delamater AM, Jacobson, AM, Anderson, BJ, *et al.* Psychosocial therapies in diabetes: report of the Psychosocial Therapies Working Group. *Diabetes Care.* 2001; **24**(7): 1286–92.

Delamater AM, Kurtz SM, White NH, *et al.* Effects of social demand on reports of self-monitored blood glucose in adolescents with type 1 diabetes mellitus. *J Appl Soc Psychol* 1988; **18**(1): 491–502.

Diabetes Control and Complications Trial Research Group (DCCT). Effect of intensive diabetes treatment on the development and progression of long-term complications in adolescents with insulin-dependent diabetes mellitus, Diabetes Control and Complications Trial. *J Pediatr.* 1994; **125**(2): 177–88.

Ellis DA, Podolski C, Frey M, *et al.* The role of parental monitoring in adolescent health outcomes: impact of regimen adherence in youth with type 1 diabetes. *J Pediatr Psychol.* 2007; **32**(8): 907–17.

Hains AA, Berlin KS, Davies WH. Attributions of adolescents with type 1 diabetes related to performing diabetes care around friends and peers: the moderating role of friend support. *J Pediatr Psychol.* 2007; **32**(5): 561–70.

Hanson CL, Cigrant JA, Harris M, *et al.* Coping styles in youths with insulin-dependent diabetes mellitus. *J Consult Clin Psychol.* 1989; **57**(5): 644–51.

Hauser S, Jacobson A, Lavori P, *et al.* Adherence among children and adolescents with insulin dependent diabetes mellitus over a four year longitudinal follow-up: II. Immediate and long-term linkages with the family milieu. *J Pediatr Psychol.* 1990; **15**(4): 527–42.

Haynes RB, Taylor DW, Sackett DL. *Compliance in Health Care.* Baltimore, MD: Johns Hopkins University Press; 1979.

Helgeson VS, Reynolds KA, Siminerio L, *et al.* Parent and adolescent distribution of responsibility for diabetes self care. *J Pediatr Psychol.* 2008; **33**(5): 497–508.

Helgeson VS, Snyder PR, Escobar O, *et al.* Comparison of adolescents with and without diabetes on indices of psychosocial functioning for three years. *J Pediatr Psychol.* 2007; **32**(7): 794–806.

Jacobson A, Hauser ST, Lavori P, *et al.* Adherence among children and adolescents with insulin dependent diabetes mellitus over a four year longitudinal follow-up: I. The influence of patient coping and adjustment. *J Pediatr Psychol.* 1990; **15**(4): 511–52.

Jacobson AM, Hauser ST, Willett J, *et al.* Consequences of irregular versus continuous medical follow-up in children and adolescents with insulin-dependent diabetes mellitus. *J Pediatr.* 1997; **131**(5): 727–33.

Johnson SB, Kelly M, Henretta JC, *et al.* A longitudinal analysis of adherence and health status in childhood diabetes. *J Pediatr Psychol.* 1992; **17**(5): 537–53.

Kovacs M, Goldston D, Obrosky DS, *et al.* Prevalence and predictors of pervasic non-compliance with medical treatment among youths with insulin-dependent diabetes mellitus. *J Am Acad Child Adolesc Psychiatry.* 1992; **31**(6): 1112–19.

Kurtz, SMS. Adherence to diabetes regimen: empirical status and clinical applications. *Diabetes Educ.* 1990; **16**(1); 50–6.

Kyngäs HA. Predictors of good adherence of adolescents with diabetes (insulin-dependent diabetes mellitus). *Chronic Illn.* 2007; **3**(1): 20–8.

La Greca AM, Bearman KJ, Moore H. Peer relations of youth with pediatric conditions and health risks: promoting social support and healthy lifestyles. *J Dev Behav Pediatr.* 2002; **23**(4): 271–80.

La Greca AM, Mackey ER. Adherence to pediatric treatment regimens. In: Roberts MC, Steele RG, editors. *Handbook of Pediatric Psychology.* New York, NY: Guilford Press; 2009. pp. 130–52.

Lewandowski A, Drotar D. The relationship between parent-reported social support and adherence to medical treatment in families of adolescents with type 1 diabetes. *J Pediatr Psychol.* 2007; **32**(4): 427–36.

Littlefield CH, Craven JL, Rodin GM, *et al.* Relationship of self-efficacy and binging to adherence to diabetes regimen among adolescents. *Diabetes Care.* 1992; **15**(1): 90–4.

McGrady M, Laffel L, Drotar D, *et al.* Depression and glycemic control in adolescents with type 1 diabetes: mediational role of adherence. *Diabetes Care.* 2009; **32**(5): 804–6.

Meichenbaum D, Turk DC. *Facilitating Treatment Adherence: a practitioner's guidebook.* New York, NY: Plenum Press; 1987.

Miller-Johnson S, Emery R, Marvin R, *et al.* Parent-child relationships and the management of insulin-dependent diabetes mellitus. *J Consult Clin Psychol.* 1994; **62**(3): 603–10.

Murphy L, Thompson RJ, Morris MA. Adherence behavior among adolescents with type 1 insulin dependent diabetes: the role of cognitive processes. *J Pediatr Psychol.* 1997; **22**(6): 811–25.

Naar-King S, Podolski CL, Ellis DA, *et al.* Social ecological model of illness management in high risk youths with type 1 diabetes. *J Consult Clin Psychol.* 2006; **74**(4): 785–9.

Neumark-Sztainer D, Patterson J, Mellin A, *et al.* Weight control practices and disordered eating behaviors among adolescent females and males with type 1 diabetes: associations with sociodemographics, weight concerns, familial factors, and metabolic outcomes. *Diabetes Care.* 2002; **25**(8): 1289–96.

Quittner, A, Modi, A, Lemanek, K, *et al.* Evidence-based assessment of adherence to medical treatments in pediatric psychology. *J Pediatr Psychol.* 2007; **33**(9): 916–36.

Reynolds L, Johnson SB, Silverstein J. Assessing daily diabetes management by 24-hour recall interview: the validity of children's report. *J Pediatr Psychol.* 1990; **15**(4): 493–510.

Schmidt LE, Klover RV, Arfken CL, *et al.* Compliance with dietary prescriptions in children and adolescents with insulin-dependent diabetes mellitus. *J Am Diet Assoc.* 1992; **92**(5): 567–70.

Skinner TC, John M, Hampson SE. Social support and personal models of diabetes as predictors of self care and well-being: a longitudinal study of adolescents with diabetes. *J Pediatr Psychol.* 2000; **25**(4): 257–67.

Thomas AM, Peterson L, Goldstein D. Problem solving and diabetes regimen adherence by children and adolescents with IDDM in social pressure situations: a reflection of normal development. *J Pediatr Psychol.* 1997; **22**(4): 541–61.

Weissberg-Benchell J, Glasgow AM, Tynan WD, *et al.* Adolescent management and mismanagement. *Diabetes Care.* 1995; **18**(1): 77–82.

Wysocki T, Iannotti R, Weissberg-Benchell J, *et al.* Diabetes problem solving by youths with Type 1 diabetes and their caregivers: measurement, validation and longitudinal associations with glycemic control. *J Pediatr Psychol.* 2008; **33**(8): 875–84.

Wysocki T, Taylor A, Hough B, *et al.* Deviation from developmentally appropriate self-care autonomy: association with diabetes outcomes. *Diabetes Care.* 1996; **19**(2): 119–25.

CHAPTER 5

The effects of diabetes on cognitive function

Angela Griffin and Deborah Christie

INTRODUCTION

There are a number of diabetes-related variables that have the potential to impact on brain development and, as a consequence, on neuropsychological functioning. These variables operate independently of one another and have different pathological mechanisms. The young brain is a dynamic organism with specific structural and functional developments occurring at predetermined times and, as with any brain insult, the consequences vary depending on the timing. Early age at the onset of diabetes and a history of severe hypoglycaemia have emerged as the most consistent predictors of adverse neuropsychological effects in children. Hyperglycaemia effects have been more difficult to investigate, as HbA_{1c} is the most commonly used index and this provides only a 2- to 3-month record of metabolic control.

Overall differences in intellectual functioning between diabetes groups and controls tend to be small, with most children continuing to function within the average range. However, the differences are substantial enough to impact on learning in the classroom, and it is likely that the cohorts studied include some children who do significantly more poorly. The subtle nature of the differences also means that children's difficulties are at greater risk of being overlooked (Gaudieri *et al.*, 2008; Naguib *et al.*, 2009).

This chapter has two sections: the first section presents the current research, including consideration of the impact of diabetes variables on cognitive function and the mechanism of effects; the second section outlines the impact of difficulties on day-to-day functioning, how to spot them and what kinds of strategies will help children to maximise their potential.

RESEARCH ISSUES

Historically, much of the evidence regarding the impact of childhood diabetes on cognitive function was derived from research with adults (Rovet, 2000). Attempts to extrapolate the findings from adult diabetes research downwards to apply them to children is problematic because of the effects of historical variables, such as response to treatment, changes in diabetes management and how these interact with maturation.

Research with children has faced its own challenges. It has been characterised by small sample sizes, the use of retrospective accounts of hypoglycaemia and imprecise definitions of physical status such as 'severe hypoglycaemia', making comparison and interpretation difficult. Understanding the impact of abnormal glycaemic levels is hampered by methodological considerations. The vast majority of evidence regarding the long-term effects of hypoglycaemia on neuropsychological functioning is based on adults with longstanding diabetes and the results are controversial (Rovet, 2000). Adequate controls are often lacking. Studies that use sibling control groups are problematic because of a similar heritability risk for learning difficulties that can confound disease-related performance difference (Lavigne, 1979). Equally many studies are cross-sectional, which restricts understanding of potential causality. In contrast, longitudinal assessment starting at an early age can also create challenges, as psychometric tests change as children grow older and therefore comparability over time is restricted. Finally, studies focus on different cognitive domains and use different tests to measure supposedly similar skills. Two recent meta-analyses (Gaudieri et al., 2008; Naguib et al., 2009) have gone some way towards synthesising the most reliable findings to date.

Gaudieri et al.'s (2008) meta-analysis of 19 studies reported that children with diabetes performed slightly less well than controls on verbal and non-verbal intelligence and specific skills such as attention and executive function. Comparison between children with diabetes and those without revealed core differences in all broad cognitive domains (except learning and memory). Children with early-onset diabetes (before age 7) were more adversely affected than those with late onset. Learning and memory skills were on average half a standard deviation lower in early-onset children than in the non-diabetes control group, which is likely to be detectable in performance in the classroom. The late-onset group showed slight but detectable performance decrements compared with the control group on visual learning and memory, visual motor integration and psychomotor speed. Academic achievement was also slightly lower for early-onset children than for late-onset children and children in the control group. Overall, there is a degree of consensus that early-onset diabetes creates moderate cognitive deficits in children, with particularly negative effects on memory and learning. While it is reported that seizures are related to nominal inconsistent performance differences, Gaudieri *et al.* (2008) do not comment further on the effects of specific disease-related variables.

Naguib *et al.* (2009) established a generic classification system so that all relevant studies could be included in their meta-analysis of 24 studies, despite the differences in psychometric tools used. The classification system provides a useful overview of the range of cognitive skills that have been assessed in different research projects. The seven cognitive areas that emerge are (i) general intelligence, (ii) visuospatial skills, (iii) language and education, (iv) memory and learning, (v) psychomotor activity, (vi) attention and (vii) executive function.

They found a significant impact on sustained attention, visuospatial ability, motor speed, writing and reading. Consistent with Gaudieri *et al.* (2008), children with diabetes also showed a reduction in verbal and non-verbal intelligence. While these reductions are small, they place children at a disadvantage in relation to peers, especially in demanding academic environments. Non-verbal intellectual abilities are particularly vulnerable to the effects of early-onset diabetes. Naguib *et al.* (2009) suggested that this is probably accounted for by the vulnerability of perceptual skills to early childhood brain insult (Taylor and Alden, 1997) and the greater impact of diffuse diabetes-related metabolic changes on the young brain (Davis *et al.*, 2002; Schoenle *et al.*, 2002). It has been suggested that reduced motor speed may be the childhood equivalent of the slowing of mental ability found in adult studies (Brands *et al.*, 2005). The visuospatial anomalies, reduced motor speed and sustained attention effects may underpin subsequent difficulties with reading and writing. Severe hypoglycaemic attacks were also found to be associated with small but significant effects on short-term verbal memory.

While the meta-analyses provide a useful overview of the research findings, they do not thoroughly address the relationship between specific disease variables and associated cognitive effects. The current evidence is presented here.

CLINICAL VARIABLES

Hypoglycaemia and seizures

Intensive treatment regimens, while reducing HbA_{1c} and the microvascular consequences of diabetes, have the side effect of causing higher incidence of hypoglycaemic events (DCCT, 1993). Approximately 31% of children with type 1 diabetes experience hypoglycaemia at some point, owing to the difficulty in balancing insulin injections with activity and diet in a growing child (Daneman, 1989). As very young children may be unable to identify symptoms or to verbalise them, and as activity levels are harder to predict, they are at greater risk of severe hypoglycaemic episodes (Eeg-Olofsson, 1966). This is especially problematic, as the early years are also the time of most rapid brain development. Neurologically, it is a time of both opportunity and vulnerability, with critical periods for the development of various skills and abilities. Ryan (2004) argues that hypoglycaemic episodes affect neuropsychological function selectively in children with early-onset diabetes (diagnosed before they are 6 years old). This is because the first 5 years of life are thought to be an especially critical period for brain development, with a special sensitivity to changes in glucose levels potentially resulting in an enhanced likelihood of structural and functional brain and neurocognitive deficits in this age group.

However, there is limited evidence about which specific hypoglycaemia-related variables are particularly important in determining the potentially adverse effects on the developing brain. The hippocampus, which contains the most insulin receptors, may be most adversely affected by hypoglycaemia. As the hippocampus is principally associated with learning and memory, it is suggested that these are the abilities most likely to be affected (Hershey *et al.*, 1997). However, studies also examined specific effects on a broad range of abilities, such as motor speed, visuospatial skills, attention, memory and executive function.

Hannonen *et al.* (2003) compared children with and without a history of severe hypoglycaemia and children without diabetes aged between 5 and 12 years. The group with severe hypoglycaemia showed more neuropsychological impairments than the other two groups, with significant differences in short-term verbal memory and phonological processing – two skill areas with the potential to impact significantly on literacy and learning. However, the diabetes group without severe hypoglycaemia also had slightly poorer auditory-verbal skills than the children without diabetes. They also differed in a task requiring executive function skills. Hannonen *et al.* (2003) argue that this may be due to the mild symptomatic or asymptomatic hypoglycaemic episodes that all children with diabetes experience. These cause transient cognitive deficits, especially in planning and cognitive flexibility, sustained attention and reaction time (Ryan, 1990) and may have a cumulative, negative effect on the child's performance. This would support a view that diabetes causes subtle, diffuse deficits in performance (Hannonen *et al.*, 2003).

In contrast, Strudwick *et al.* (2005) failed to find evidence of general cognitive dysfunction or specific memory deficits in 41 children under 6 years old with a history of hypoglycaemic-related seizure or coma compared with a control group of children with diabetes but without a history of severe hypoglycaemia. Rovet *et al.* (1988) and Ryan *et al.* (1985) also found no correlation between hypoglycaemia and cognitive test scores, although both studies used HbA$_{1c}$ alone as an indicator of metabolic control. Northam *et al.* (1992) suggest that perhaps a longer-term measure of poor control is necessary before associations become apparent.

It has also been argued that children diagnosed early may have more seizures because of the behavioural and medical challenges of disease management in young children. Therefore, early onset may mask the possible underlying effects of seizures. However, Gaudieri *et al.* (2008) suggest that the effects of seizures are more benign than thought and are not a surrogate for early-onset effects and that interactive or synergistic effects are more likely, if anything. Seizures were related to the smallest overall cognitive effects. These effects may be greater for children who have chronic poor metabolic control and who have been shown to have lower scores on psychometric tests in individual studies.

TABLE 5.1 Effects of hypoglycaemia on cognitive function

Authors	Study group	Cognitive effects
Ryan *et al.* (1985)	Type 1 diabetes mellitus (T1DM) (n = 125), non-T1DM (n = 83)	Using most recent HbA$_{1c}$ level, no relationship between hypoglycaemia and cognitive test scores found
Rovet *et al.* (1988)	27 children with early onset of diabetes (EOD < 4 year), 24 children with late onset of diabetes (LOD > 4 year) and 30 siblings as control	Older children with later disease onset began to evidence a minor decline in verbal functioning
Rovet and Alvarez (1997)	Type 1 diabetes mellitus (T1DM) (n = 103) Non-T1DM (n = 100)	History of hypoglycaemia and hypoglycaemic seizures associated with lower verbal IQ scores and lower scores on aspects of attention
Rovet and Ehrlich (1999)	T1DM (n = 16) assessed at diagnosis and 1, 3 and 7 years post-diagnosis	At 7 years post-diagnosis, reduction in verbal skills but not visuospatial skills
Hannonen *et al.* (2003)	T1DM and severe hypo (n = 11) T1DM without severe hypo (n = 10) Non-T1DM controls (n = 10)	Short-term verbal memory and phonological processing worse in severe hypo group than in other two groups. Poorer auditory-verbal skills in T1DM without severe hypo group than in healthy controls. More special educational input received
Strudwick *et al.* (2005)	< 6 years old, T1DM and severe hypo/seizures/coma (n = 41) T1DM without severe hypo (n = 43)	No significant differences between groups on intellectual, memory or behavioural measures
Gaudieri *et al.* (2008)	Meta-analysis	Effects of hypoglycaemic seizures greatest in those with chronic poor metabolic control. Otherwise, effects of seizures on cognition minimal

Authors	Study group	Cognitive effects
Northam *et al.* (2009)	T1DM (n = 106) Non-T1DM (n = 75)	At 12 years post-diagnosis, T1DM group showed lower verbal IQ and full scale IQ than baseline and non-T1DM
		Lower verbal IQ associated with history of hypoglycaemia and with volume reduction in thalamus

Hyperglycaemia

The Diabetes Control and Complications Trial showed that repeated hyperglycaemia associated with persistent raised HbA$_{1c}$ contributes to increased risk of complications of diabetes, including retinopathy, nephropathy and neuropathy. Extreme hyperglycaemia due to lack of insulin can cause diabetic ketoacidosis (DKA), which can lead to acute illness, loss of consciousness and even coma or death. Severe DKA may result in central nervous system damage. While it was originally thought that non-DKA episodes of hyperglycaemia were likely to have little or no effect on cognitive function, research is now beginning to suggest that there may indeed be consequences. For example, chronic hyperglycaemia may disrupt myelin formation and neurotransmitter regulation in the developing brain (Rovet and Alvarez, 1997). Rovet *et al.* (1990) used parent diaries completed retrospectively and information on hospitalisations. They found a correlation between a history of hyperglycaemia-related ketonuria and poor spatial skills 1 year after diagnosis. Kaufman *et al.* (1999) reported that children with elevated HbA$_{1c}$ levels over a 2-year period did poorly on a verbal selective reminding task, indicating difficulty in this area of memory and executive functioning. Perantie *et al.* (2008) described effects of hyperglycaemia on fine motor control tasks, with a trend for hyperglycaemia to affect more demanding motor reaction tasks. However, these results were not replicated in the same group at a later age (Rovet *et al.*, 1993) or in a study involving induced hyperglycaemia (Gschwend *et al.*, 1995). Perantie *et al.* (2008) also found hyperglycaemia specifically affected verbal intelligence.

In Perantie *et al.*'s 2008 study, hyperglycaemia was found to specifically affect verbal intelligence. Ferguson *et al.* (2003) studied young people for 10 years post-diagnosis. Chronic hyperglycaemia, inferred by the presence of diabetic retinopathy, was associated with poorer performance on cognitive tests of fluid (spatial) intelligence, information processing speed and sustained attention.

Rovet and Alvarez (1997) subsequently identified an association between high blood glucose levels and difficulty with executive function tasks that required inhibition skills.

TABLE 5.2 Effects of hyperglycaemia on cognitive function

Authors	Study group	Cognitive effects
Rovet et al. (1988)	Type 1 diabetes mellitus (T1DM) children (n = 103) Healthy controls (n = 100)	Induced concurrent hyperglycaemia associated with drop in executive function skill of inhibition
Rovet et al. (1990)	Parent diaries of episodes of hypo-/ hyperglycaemia and hospitalisations	History of ketonuria caused by hyperglycaemia related to poor spatial skills at 1 year post-diagnosis
Kaufman et al. (1999)	55 of 62 eligible children with diabetes (mean age 7.9 +/− 1.6 years) matched with 15 siblings acting as controls	Children with elevated HbA_{1c} in 2 years prior performed poorly on verbal selective reminding tests
Ferguson et al. (2003)	Cross-sectional study of 74 young people with T1DM	Chronic hyperglycaemia related to poorer spatial intelligence, information processing speed and sustained attention
Perantie et al. (2008)	T1DM children aged 5–16 years (n = 117) Non-diabetic sibling controls (n = 58)	Verbal intelligence and demanding motor reaction tasks adversely affected by increased exposure to hyperglycaemia

Individual variables
Age at onset of diabetes
Attempts have been made to map the developmental trajectory of cognitive risk in diabetes and to examine the interaction between onset and frequency or duration of exposure to glycaemic extremes on selected cognitive functions. Perantie *et al.* (2008) found that hypo- and hyperglycaemia had different effects on cognitive function, determined partly by the amount of exposure during development but not by the age of onset. Studies found that verbal intelligence was reduced in those with increased exposure to hyperglycaemia, while spatial intelligence and delayed recall were reduced following repeated hypoglycaemia, especially when episodes began before the age of 5 years.

However, research findings on the impact of duration of diabetes are ambiguous. In a population of children and young people, duration will often be confounded by early onset, which in itself is related to cognitive outcome. Fox *et al.* (2003) found that the most potent predictor of learning was disease duration, followed by gender. The interaction between duration of diabetes and gender was not a significant performance predictor, suggesting that cumulative and chronic exposure to the metabolic abnormalities typical of diabetes alone is a major risk factor related to poorer learning over time. However, Perantie *et al.* (2008) argued that duration of diabetes per se was not associated with lower verbal intelligence or with performance on memory tasks.

Gender

Evidence of a greater impact on learning in boys diagnosed with diabetes fits with the neurodevelopmental literature of greater vulnerability of the male brain, thought to be due to foetal surges in androgens (Geschwind and Galaburda, 1985; Juraska, 1986), as well as testosterone-induced changes in the structure of the hypothalamus and limbic systems, areas associated with memory and learning.

In Fox *et al.*'s 2003 study, boys aged 11–15 years with diabetes failed to make developmental gains on a verbal learning task compared with boys without diabetes and compared with girls with or without diabetes. This failure to learn more at the follow-up test occurred during a period of rapid growth and maturation, when volume and speed of acquisition of new material should increase substantially (Gitomer and Pellegrino, 1985). Remembering information from the first part of a list was particularly affected (primacy learning). Boys with diabetes have also shown decreasing vocabulary scores over an 8-year period (Kovacs and Ryan, 1994) and a decline in cued learning over a 6-year period (Northam *et al.*, 2001). Boys also do less well than girls with diabetes or controls on tasks requiring auditory attention and verbal memory, and they show more general learning problems than other groups (Holmes *et al.*, 1992).

Finally, boys may also lose their gender advantage on spatial tasks. Holmes *et al.* (1992) reported that boys with diabetes performed worse than those without diabetes on visuospatial tasks and in fact they performed the same as girls with or without diabetes.

Social and cultural factors

Soutor *et al.* (2004) found that ethnicity only accounts for 3% of the variance in blood glucose monitoring in adolescents. Hassan *et al.* (2006) found higher socio-economic status was associated with better glycaemic control and quality of life. Overstreet *et al.* (1997) found that while boys tend to perform more poorly than girls on tests of verbal learning, higher socio-economic status appears to provide some protection for boys.

MECHANISM OF IMPACT ON THE DEVELOPING BRAIN

Developmental course

The brain is thought to be particularly vulnerable to the effects of hypoglycaemia during the neonatal period. Preterm infants born small for gestational age (Lucas *et al.*, 1988), infants of mothers with diabetes (Schwartz and Teramo, 2000) and infants with persistent hyperinsulinaemic hypoglycaemia (Cresto *et al.*, 1998) are most at risk. Neurodevelopmental outcome can be affected even after moderate neonatal hypoglycaemia (Lucas *et al.*, 1988), and prolonged or repeated episodes of profound neonatal hypoglycaemia may lead to severe learning disability and epilepsy (Menni *et al.*, 2001).

Although children with diabetes are usually older when they experience hypoglycaemia, it appears that cognitive effects, although mild, appear relatively quickly following diagnosis (Gaudieri *et al.*, 2008). At the time of diagnosis, there are no differences between children with and without diabetes in terms of neuropsychological functioning and academic achievement (Kovacs and Ryan, 1994; Northam *et al.*, 1998). At 1-year follow-up, Rovet *et al.* (1990) still found no difference, although older children with later disease onset were beginning to show a minor decline in verbal functioning (Rovet and Ehrlich, 1999). At 2- and 6-year follow-up, Northam *et al.* (1998, 2001) found those with earlier onset showed smaller verbal gains than controls, though scores remained within the average range. Episodes of severe hypoglycaemia significantly predicted lower verbal IQ at 6-year follow-up.

Perantie *et al.* (2008) suggest that hypoglycaemia experienced early in development is more harmful to neural systems underlying delayed memory than hypoglycaemia later in life. In a retrospective study, they found that age of exposure to hypoglycaemic events was related to reduced verbal and visual delayed recall and spatial intelligence, rather than age at onset of diabetes per se.

Puberty is considered an independent risk factor for the complications of diabetes because of the increased insulin resistance associated with gonadal and adrenal hormone changes at this time (Bloch *et al.*, 1987; Caprio *et al.*, 1989), which may lead to increased risk of hyperglycaemia. Hyperglycaemia has been shown to affect the timing of myelination (Vlassara *et al.*, 1983). The frontal lobes and parts of the reticular formation have a protracted period of myelination that continues on into the teens and twenties, and these structures may be vulnerable to episodes of hyperglycaemia during puberty (Yakovlev and Lecours, 1975).

Rovet and Ehrlich (1999) noted executive function deficits in adolescents with diabetes, regardless of the age of onset. Those who developed diabetes during later childhood and adolescence also showed poorer scores on tests of vocabulary and general knowledge (Ryan *et al.*, 1984).

Desrocher and Rovet (2004) have proposed a timeline model of the relationship between diabetes variables and neurocognitive development. This links the age-related development of specific brain areas with the skills these areas underpin, as well as with the diabetes variables most likely to be impacting at that time. The brain areas responsible for the development of motor, sensory and visuospatial function are developing most rapidly in the child's preschool years, and so these skills are most likely to be affected by hypoglycaemia, which is usually a feature of early-onset diabetes. The parietal lobes experience a critical period of development in the early school years. This means that visuospatial skills and attentional processes increase in complexity. The hippocampus undergoes rapid development between the ages of 7 and 12 years, enabling expansion and increasing complexity in memory functioning. Throughout these years, hypoglycaemia has the potential to impact on the brain, and these developing areas may be particularly vulnerable. As the prefrontal cortex develops in the adolescent period, young people develop planning and organisational skills necessary for increasing independence and more sophisticated thinking. Hyperglycaemia is most likely to be prevalent in this age category and to have an adverse impact on these specific skills. While brain development is not quite as linear as this in real life, the model may provide a basis for research into connections between brain development during critical periods and the adverse effects of specific diabetes variables.

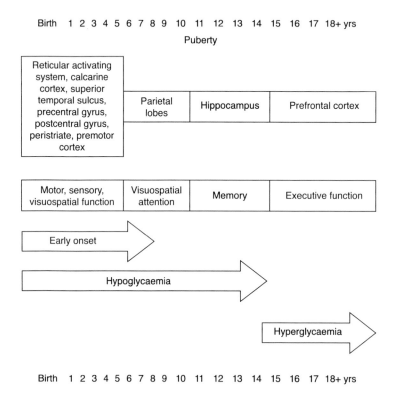

FIGURE 5.1 Relationship between diabetes variables and neurocognitive development

NEUROPATHOLOGY: SPECIFIC VERSUS DIFFUSE

Glucose is the major energy source for the brain, and optimal levels of circulating glucose are necessary for normal neuronal functioning (Holmes, 1986). Children's brains may be more sensitive to glucose fluctuation, as they have high cerebral energy requirements related to rapid brain growth and neural pruning (Northam *et al.*, 2009). Chalmers *et al.* (1991) reported that abnormal blood glucose levels particularly affect the frontal and temporal regions of the brain, especially the hippocampus. The frontal and temporal regions, especially in the left hemisphere, are involved in language, memory and attentional processes. Hypoglycaemic conditions may also have adverse effects on attention, executive function, learning and memory. Subtle changes in electrical measurements of brain activity have been described, even in those only recently diagnosed with diabetes (Cirilo *et al.*, 1984; Donald *et al.*, 1984).

In a longitudinal study, Northam *et al.* (2009) reported that hypoglycaemia was associated with lower verbal IQ and volume reduction in the thalamus at 12 years post-diagnosis. Strong associations were also found between older age and reduced volume in anterior and temporal brain regions, as well as the thalamus, caudate and lentiform nuclei. As the same group has been followed over a 12-year period, older age is a surrogate for later disease onset in this study. The link between older age at onset and volume reductions is surprising, given the consistent association between early disease onset and cognitive deficits. Northam *et al.* (2009) suggest that it may reflect an interaction between diabetes and the final stages of neurodevelopment, which continue into the third decade of life. It may be that the younger group is yet to experience these effects. Ferguson (2005) also found that individuals with early-onset disease had larger ventricular volumes and more prevalent ventricular atrophy than those with later onset, which corresponded to poorer intellectual and information processing ability.

In animal studies, Yamada *et al.* (2004) have reported that moderate hypoglycaemia in a developing rat brain can result in neuronal death in the cortex and disruption of the neural activity linked to learning in the hippocampus. Hypoglycaemia also exacerbates an increase in cortisol levels, which decreases hippocampal size. Early exposure to hypoglycaemia may therefore disrupt the development of connections within the hippocampus and/or between the hippocampus and cortex (Saykin *et al.*, 1989; Lipska *et al.*, 2002).

Alterations in cerebral blood flow and biochemical disturbances in the central nervous system have been described in adult patients with diabetes (Mooradian, 1988). In cerebral blood-flow studies, hypoglycaemia has been shown to have an asymmetrical effect with a greater reduction of left- versus right-hemisphere perfusion (Jarjour *et al.*, 1995), which is more marked in boys than in girls. Men have been shown to experience hypoglycaemia at higher blood glucose levels than women and correspondingly to have greater cognitive disruption than women during hypoglycaemia (Gonder-Frederick *et al.*, 1994). This would suggest it is important for boys to avoid even mild hypoglycaemia, especially when at school.

Hyperglycaemia is known to disrupt blood–brain barrier function and reduce cerebral blood flow acutely, while chronic hyperglycaemia is connected to cerebrovascular disease and neuropathy (McCall and Figleqicz, 1997). Chronic hyperglycaemia may disrupt metabolite levels (Northam *et al.*, 2009), myelin formation and neurotransmitter regulation in the developing brain (Rovet and Alvarez, 1997). Increased levels of metabolites (myoinositol and choline) are related to demyelination and other types of cell membrane breakdown, such as gliosis. In Northam *et al.*'s 2009 12-year follow-up study, poorer metabolic control was associated with higher levels of myoinositol and choline in frontal and temporal lobes and in the basal ganglia. Cameron *et al.* (2005) found elevated myoinositol in children recovering from DKA. Northam *et al.* (2009) suggest this may indicate that higher metabolite levels may represent a homeostatic response of the brain to prolonged hyperglycaemia. N-acetylaspartate (NAA) is a marker for neuronal density, and lower levels indicate neuronal death or decreased neuronal metabolism. NAA levels have been found to correlate inversely with hyperglycaemia (Makimattila *et al.*, 2004), and animal studies have shown that chronic hyperglycaemia reduces neuronal number and impedes myelination (Malone *et al.*, 2006). Northam *et al.* (2009) found that subjects with diabetes had lower NAA in the frontal lobes and basal ganglia. Metabolite profiles have not been found to be related to a history of hypoglycaemia (Northam *et al.*, 2009).

Biessels *et al.* (2006) have proposed that the changes found in the brains of those with diabetes may represent an 'accelerated ageing' trajectory. This implies that rather than changes being associated with disrupted neurodevelopment, the volume loss detected in those who are older or who had later onset of diabetes represent the early stages of neurodegeneration or microvascular disease.

Impact on functioning at school

Although boys and girls with diabetes have been reported to achieve intelligence quotient scores in the average to high-average ranges, the group average has been found to be three to seven points lower than that of a control group (Holmes *et al.*, 1992). These mild difficulties may have a cumulative effect, and in particular they may create subtle difficulties for specific groups of children.

It is unclear whether the impact on intelligence, memory and other cognitive functions is reflected in everyday cognitive, social or academic functioning. However, even minor problems in neurocognitive functioning can cause learning difficulties at school. As previously described, mild hypoglycaemic episodes have an influence on attention (Ryan 1990; Gschwend *et al.*, 1995), psychomotor speed and memory (Reich *et al.*, 1990). Teachers may not be aware that a child is experiencing hypoglycaemic attention difficulties and so may fail to provide appropriate support.

Ryan (1988) reported poorer school achievement among children with diabetes, especially in reading and spelling. Hannonen *et al.* (2003) reported that children with diabetes, and especially those who had experienced severe hypoglycaemia, had more learning difficulties reported by parents and needed more part-time special education than unaffected children. Holmes *et al.* (1992) found that up to one third of boys with diabetes are reported by their parents to have had learning difficulties at some point in their school career. Seventeen per cent received a formal diagnosis of learning difficulty or hyperactivity, and 29% had resource room instruction at some point. Forty per cent of the boys with diabetes had had special input, repeated a school year, or both. Four per cent of girls had repeated a year and 12% had special intervention. The number of girls receiving special instruction was double that of those without diabetes, suggesting diabetes had an impact on the school performance of both girls and boys (Holmes *et al.*, 1992). Fowler *et al.* (1985) reported that in terms of academic functioning, children with diabetes do more poorly than healthy children and only those children with a neurological illness, e.g. epilepsy, are more adversely affected.

Even if studies do not find statistical differences between children and young people with diabetes and normal controls, there may still be both direct and indirect effects on day-to-day functioning that become apparent over time (Strudwick *et al.*, 2005). Therefore, it is essential to monitor and detect intra-individual change rather than relying on large-scale group differences. It is also important to make sure that while there may be progress over time, it is sufficient and adequate.

PRESENTING SYMPTOMS IN THE CLASSROOM

The potentially adverse effect of diabetes on verbal memory has been outlined by a number of longitudinal research studies (Fox *et al.*, 2003; Kovacs and Ryan, 1994; Northam *et al.*, 2001). As verbal memory is increasingly critical in the school years (Schneider and Pressley, 1989), this may have a marked impact on learning. The impact of these cognitive effects may also extend to managing the diabetes regimen, which has significant memory demands. While some of these are relatively simple, repetitive tasks, such as blood glucose monitoring, others require more complex memory skills, such as ongoing carbohydrate counting and calculation of insulin-correction doses throughout the day. In adolescents who are likely to be asked to take increasing responsibility for their treatment, the demands on memory will be greater. As mentioned earlier, adolescence is a key time for the development of organisation and planning skills and is therefore a time of maximum vulnerability to the disruption of the skills that will be essential in managing the complexity of diabetes self-care. Soutor *et al.* (2004) found that quantitative working memory is the only significant predictor of carbohydrates consumed. This indicates that remembering and calculating continual daily carbohydrate consumption is a complex task that is heavily memory dependent. They also found that verbal memory accounts for a small amount of the variance in daily blood glucose tests. Memory can be enhanced through the use of compensatory strategies and environmental supports (Schneider and Pressley, 1989), and this may be a useful addition to clinical treatment.

Identifying difficulties with working memory and providing remediation and support for this could therefore potentially offset the decline in self-care skills typically occurring during adolescence (Wysocki, 1990). As diabetes management becomes more personalised but more complex, the focus may also extend to other cognitive skills such as problem-solving and cognitive flexibility, which will be needed if self-care is to be optimised (*see* Part III).

SUMMARY

As described in previous chapters, the majority of children and young people with diabetes fail to achieve adequate metabolic control. As a result, their developing brains are vulnerable to frank neurological insult through hypoglycaemia and hyperglycaemia, and DKA Healthcare teams, teachers, parents and young people should be aware of the potential cognitive vulnerability associated with hypoglycaemic seizures and chronic hyperglycaemia. Early detection of minor difficulties should be a priority. Assessment of cognitive skills is as essential as teaching carbohydrate counting and insulin dose adjustment, as it will impact on the day-to-day management of diabetes.

Early onset of diabetes is associated with the greatest impact on cognitive function in children. It is unclear whether the association is because of the high risk of recurrent severe hypoglycaemia in young children. Longer disease duration is another predictor of impairment. Further research that incorporates pathophysiological measures, cognitive measures and measure of daily functioning on a longitudinal basis is needed. While frank hypoglycaemia and hyperglycaemia are currently targeted in research, improvement in continuous glucose monitoring may allow for the inclusion of asymptomatic or nocturnal hypoglycaemia as further disease variables that may contribute to cognitive difficulties.

Teacher reports play a key role in the ability to investigate the links between assessment results and day-to-day functioning. Rigorous longitudinal (as opposed to cross-sectional) studies with continuous glucose monitoring systems to track glucose excursions may better examine the progression of cognitive functioning over time. It is important to monitor children with diabetes to ensure that subtle learning difficulties identified (Rovet *et al.*, 1990, 1997; Northam *et al.*, 1998, 2001) do not take a cumulative educational or psychological toll.

REFERENCES

Austin E, Deary I. Effects of repeated hypoglycemia on cognitive function: a psychometrically validated reanalysis of the diabetes control and complications trial data. *Diabetes Care.* 1999; **22**(8): 1273–7.

Biessels G, Staekenborg S, Brunner E, *et al.* Risk of dementia in diabetes mellitus: a systematic review. *Lancet Neurol.* 2006; **5**(1): 64–74.

Brands A, Biessels G, De Haan E, *et al.* The effects of type 1 diabetes on cognitive performance. *Diabetes Care.* 2005; **288**(6): 728–37.

Bjorgaas M, Gimse R, Vik T, *et al.* Cognitive function in type 1 diabetic children with and without episodes of severe hypoglycaemia. *Acta Paediatr.* 1997; **86**(2): 148–53.

Bloch CA, Clemons P, Sperling MA. Puberty decreases insulin sensitivity. *J Pediatr.* 1987; **110**(3): 481–7.

Cameron F, Kean M, Wellard R, *et al.* Insights into the acute metabolic changes associated with childhood diabetes. *Diabet Med.* 2005; **22**(5): 648–53.

Caprio S, Plewe G, Diamond MP, *et al.* Increased insulin secretion in puberty: a compensatory response to reductions in insulin sensitivity. *J Pediatr.* 1989; **114**(6): 963–7.

Chalmers J, Risk MTA, Kean DM, *et al.* Severe amnesia after hypoglycaemia: clinical, psychometric and magnetic resonance imaging correlations. *Diabetes Care.* 1991; **14**(10): 922–5.

Cirilo D, Gonfiantini E, *et al.* Visual evoked potentials in diabetic children and adolescents. *Diabetes Care.* 1984; **7**(3): 273–5.

Cresto JC, Abdenur JP, Bergada I, *et al.* Long term follow up of persistent hyperinsulinaemic hypoglycaemia of infancy. *Arch Dis Child.* 1998; **79**(5): 440–4.

Daneman D, Frank M, Perlman K, *et al.* Severe hypoglycaemia in children with insulin-dependent diabetes mellitus: frequency and predisposing factors. *J Pediatr.* 1989; **115** (5 Pt 1): 740–2.

Davis E, Trundle C, Ives J, *et al.* High prevalence of structural central nervous system abnormalities in children with early onset diabetes. *Diabetes.* 2002; **53**(Suppl.1): A3.

Department for Education and Skills. *Every Child Matters: change for children.* Green Paper. UK: HM Government; 2003.

Desrocher M, Rovet J. Neurocognitive correlates of type 1 diabetes mellitus in childhood. *Child Neuropsychol.* 2004; **10**(1): 36–52.

Diabetes Control and Complications Trial Research Group (DCCT). The effect of intensive treatment of diabetes on the development and progression of long-term complications in insulin-dependent diabetes mellitus. *N Engl J Med.* 1993; **329**(14): 977–86.

Donald MW, Erdah D, Surridge D, *et al.* Functional correlates of reduced central conduction velocity in diabetic subjects. *Diabetes.* 1984; **33**(7): 627–33.

Eeg-Olofsson O, Petersen I. Childhood diabetic neuropathy: a clinical and neuropsychological study. *Acta Pediatr Scand.* 1966; **55**: 163–76.

Ferguson S, Blane A, Perros P, *et al.* Cognitive ability and brain structure in type 1 diabetes:

relation to microangiopathy and preceding severe hypoglycaemia. *Diabetes.* 2003; **52**(1): 149–56.

Ferguson S, Blane A, Wardlaw J, *et al.* Influence of an early-onset age of type 1 diabetes on cerebral structure and cognitive function. *Diabetes Care.* 2005; **28**(6): 1431–7.

Fowler M, Johnson M, Atkinson S. School achievement and absence in children with chronic health conditions. *J Paediatr.* 1985; **106**(4): 683–7.

Fox M, Chen R, Holmes C. Gender differences in memory and learning in children with insulin-dependent diabetes mellitus (IDDM) over a 4-year follow-up interval. *J Pediatr Psychol.* 2003; **28**(8): 569–78.

Gaudieri PA, Chen RS, Greer TF, *et al.* Cognitive function in children with type 1 diabetes: a meta-analysis. *Diabetes Care.* 2008; **31**(9): 1892–7.

Geschwind N, Galaburda A. Cerebral lateralization, biological mechanisms, associations and pathology: I. A hypothesis and a program for research. *Arch Neurol.* 1985; **42**(5): 428–59.

Gitomer D, Pellegrino J. Developmental and individual differences in long-term memory retrieval. In: Dillon RR, editor. *Individual Differences in Cognition.* Vol. 2. Orlando, FL: Academic Press; 1985. pp. 1–34.

Gonder-Frederick LA, Cox DJ, Driesen N, *et al.* Individual differences in neurobehavioral disruption during mild and moderate hypoglycemia in adults with IDDM. *Diabetes.* 1994; **43**(12): 1407–12.

Gonder-Frederick LA, Zrebiec JF, Bauchowitz AU, *et al.* Cognitive function is disrupted by both hypo- and hyperglycemia in school-aged children with type 1 diabetes: a field study. *Diabetes Care.* 2009; **32**(6): 1001–6.

Griffin A, Christie D. Taking a systemic perspective on cognitive assessments and reports. *Clin Child Psychol Psychiatry.* 2008; **13**(2): 209–20.

Gschwend S, Ryan C, Atchison J, *et al.* Effects of acute hypoglycemia on mental efficiency and counterregulatory hormones in adolescents with insulin-dependent diabetes mellitus. *J Pediatr.* 1995; **126**(2): 178–84.

Hannonen R, Tupola S, Ahonen T, *et al.* Neurocognitive functioning in children with type-1 diabetes with and without episodes of severe hypoglycaemia. *Dev Med Child Neurol.* 2003; **45**(4): 262–8.

Hassan K, Loar R, Anderson BJ, *et al.* The role of socioeconomic status, depression, quality of life, and glycemic control in type 1 diabetes mellitus. *J Pediatr.* 2006; **149**(4): 526–31.

Hershey T, Bhargava N, Sadler M, *et al.* Conventional versus intensive diabetes therapy in children with type 1 diabetes. *Diabetes Care.* 1999; **22**(8): 1318–24.

Hershey T, Craft S, Bhargava N, *et al.* Memory and insulin-dependent diabetes mellitus: effects of childhood onset and severe hypoglycaemia. *J Int Neuropsychol Soc.* 1997; **3**(6): 509–20.

Hershey T, Lillie R, Sadler M. A prospective study of severe hypoglycemia and long-term spatial memory in children with type 1 diabetes. *Pediatr Diabetes.* 2004; **5**(2): 63–71.

Hershey T, Perantie D, Warren S, *et al.* Frequency and timing of severe hypoglycemia affects spatial memory in children with type 1 diabetes. *Diabetes Care.* 2005; **28**(10): 2372–7.

Holmes CS. Neuropsychological profiles in men with insulin-dependent diabetes. *J Consult Clin Psychol.* 1986; **54**(3): 386–9.

Holmes C, Dunlap W, Chen RS, *et al.* Gender differences in the learning status of diabetic children. *J Consult Clin Psychol.* 1992; **60**(5): 698–704.

Holmes C, Richman L. Cognitive profiles of children with insulin-dependent diabetes. *J Dev Behav Pediatr.* 1985; **6**(6): 323–6.

Jarjour IT, Ryan CM, Becker DJ. Regional cerebral blood flow during hypoglycaemia in children with IDDM. *Diabetologia*. 1995; **38**(9): 1090–5.

Juraska J. Sex differences in developmental plasticity of behavior and the brain. In: Greenough WT, Jurasks JM, editors. *Developmental Neuropsychobiology*. San Diego, CA: Academic Press; 1986. pp. 409–22.

Jyothi K, Susheela S, Kodali V, *et al.* Poor cognitive task performance of insulin-dependent diabetic children (6–12 years) in India. *Diabetes Res Clin Pract*. 1993; **20**(3): 209–13.

Kaufman FR, Epport K, Engilman R, *et al.* Neurocognitive functioning in children diagnosed with diabetes before age 10 years. *J Diabetes Complications*. 1999; **13**(1): 31–8.

Kodl C, Seaquist E. Cognitive dysfunction and diabetes mellitus. *Endocr Rev*. 2008; **29**(4): 494–511.

Kovacs M, Ryan C. Verbal intellectual and verbal memory performance of youths with childhood-onset insulin-dependent diabetes mellitus. *J Pediatr Psychol*. 1994; **19**(4): 475–83.

Lavigne J, Ryan M. Psychologic adjustment to siblings of children with chronic illness. *Pediatrics*. 1979; **63**(4): 616–27.

Lipska BK, Halim ND, Segal PN, *et al.* Effects of reversible inactivation of the neonatal ventral hippocampus on behaviour in the adult rat. *J Neurosci*. 2002; **22**(7): 2835–42.

Lucas A, Morley R, Cole TJ. Adverse neurodevelopmental outcome of moderate neonatal hypoglycaemia. *BMJ*. 1988; **297**(6659): 1304–8.

Makimattila S, Malmberg-Ceder K, Hakkinen A, *et al.* Brain metabolic alterations in patients with type 1 diabetes: hyperglycemia-induced injury. *J Cereb Blood Flow Metab*. 2004; **24**(12): 1393–9.

Malone J, Hanna S, Saporta S. Hyperglycemic brain injury in the rat. *Brain Res*. 2006; **1076**(1): 9–15.

McCall A, Figleqicz D. How does diabetes mellitus produce brain dysfunctions? *Diabetes Spectrum*. 1997; **10**: 25–31.

McCarthy AM, Lindgren S, Mengeling M. Effects of diabetes on learning in children. *Pediatrics*. 2002; **109**(1): E9.

Menni F, de Lonlay P, Sevin C, *et al.* Neurologic outcomes of 90 neonates and infants with persistent hyperinsulinemic hypoglycemia. *Pediatrics*. 2001; **107**(3): 476–9.

Middleton J. Clinical neuropsychological assessment of children. In: Goldstein L, NcNeil J, editors. *Clinical Neuropsychology: a practical guide to assessment and management for clinicians*. John Wiley & Sons; 2003. pp. 275–301.

Mooradian AD. Diabetic complications of the central nervous system. *Endocr Rev*. 1988; **9**(3): 346–56.

Naguib J, Kulinskaya E, Lomax C, *et al.* Neurocognitive performance in children with type 1 diabetes: a meta-analysis. *J Pediatr Psychol*. 2009; **34**(3): 271–82.

Northam E, Anderson P, Jacobs R, *et al.* Neuropsychological profiles of children with type 1 diabetes 6 years after disease onset. *Diabetes Care*. 2001; **24**(9): 1541–6.

Northam E, Anderson P, Werther G, *et al.* Neuropsychological complications of IDDM in children 2 years after disease onset. *Diabetes Care*. 1998; **21**(3): 379–84.

Northam E, Bowden S, Anderson V, *et al.* Neuropsychological functioning in adolescents with diabetes. *J Clin Exp Neuropsychol*. 1992; **14**(6): 884–900.

Northam E, Rankins D, Lin A, *et al.* Central nervous system function in youth with type 1 diabetes 12 years after disease onset. *Diabetes Care*. 2009; **32**(3): 445–50.

Overstreet S, Holmes C, Dunlap W, *et al.* Demographic risk factors to academic and intellectual functioning in children with diabetes. *Intelligence*. 1997; **24**(2): 367–80.

Perantie D, Lim A, Wu J, *et al.* Effects of prior hypoglycemia and hyperglycemia on cognition in children with type 1 diabetes mellitus. *Pediatr Diabetes.* 2008; **9**(2): 87–95.

Reich J, Kaspar J, Puczynski M, *et al.* Effect of a hypoglycemic episode on neuropsychological functioning in children with diabetes. *J Clin Exp Neuropsychol.* 1990; **12**(4): 613–26.

Ross A, Sachdev P. Magnetic resonance spectroscopy in cognitive research. *Brain Res Rev.* 2004; **44**(2–3): 83–102.

Rovet J. Diabetes. In: Yeates KO, Ris MD, Taylor HG, editors. *Pediatric Neuropsychology, Research, Theory and Practice.* New York, NY: Guilford Press; 2000. pp. 336–65.

Rovet J, Alvarez, M. Attentional functioning in children and adolescents with IDDM. *Diabetes Care.* 1997; **20**(5): 803–10.

Rovet J, Ehrlich R. The effect of hypoglycemic seizures on cognitive function in children with diabetes: a 7-year prospective study. *J Pediatr.* 1999; **134**(4): 503–6.

Rovet J, Ehrlich R, Czuchta D. Intellectual characteristics of children with diabetes at diagnosis and one year later. *J Pediatr Psychol.* 1990; **15**(6): 775–88.

Rovet J, Ehrlich R, Czuchta D. Psychoeducational characteristics of children and adolescents with insulin-dependent diabetes mellitus. *J Learn Disabil.* 1993; **26**(1): 7–22.

Rovet J, Ehrlich R, Hoppe M. Specific intellectual deficits in children with early onset diabetes mellitus. *Child Dev.* 1988; **59**(1): 226–34.

Ryan C. Neurobehavioural complications of type 1 diabetes: examination of possible risk factors. *Diabetes Care.* 1988; **11**(1): 86–93.

Ryan C. Neuropsychological consequences and correlates of diabetes in childhood. In: Holmes CS, editor. *Neuropsychological and Behavioral Aspects of Diabetes.* New York, NY: Springer-Verlag; 1990. pp. 58–84.

Ryan C. Does moderately severe hypoglycemia cause cognitive dysfunction in children? *Pediatr Diabetes.* 2004; **5**(2): 59–62.

Ryan C, Vega A, Drash A. Cognitive deficits in adolescents who developed diabetes early in life. *Pediatrics.* 1985; **75**(5): 921–7.

Ryan C, Vega A, Longstreet C, *et al.* Neuropsychological changes in adolescents with insulin dependent diabetes. *J Consult Clin Psychol.* 1984; **52**(3): 335–42.

Schneider W, Pressley M. *Memory Development Between 2 and 20.* New York, NY: Springer-Verlag; 1989.

Schoenle E, Schoenle D, Molinari L, *et al.* Impaired intellectual development in children with type 1 diabetes: association with HbA1c, age at diagnosis and sex. *Diabetologia.* 2002; **45**(1): 108–14.

Schwartz R, Teramo KA. Effects of diabetic pregnancy on the fetus and newborn. *Semin Perinatol.* 2000; **24**(2): 120–35.

Soutor S, Rusan Chen M, Streisand R, *et al.* Memory matters: developmental differences in predictors of diabetes care behaviours. *J Pediatr Psychol.* 2004; **29**(7): 493–505.

Saykin AJ, Gur REC, Sussman NM, *et al.* Memory deficits before and after temporal lobectomy: effect of laterality and age of onset. *Brain Cogn.* 1989; **9**(2): 191–200.

Soutor S, Rusan Chen MS, Streisand R, *et al.* Memory matters: developmental differences in predictors of diabetes care behaviours. *J Pediatr Psychol.* 2004; **29**(7): 493–505.

Strudwick S, Carne C, Gardiner J, *et al.* Cognitive functioning in children with early onset type 1 diabetes and severe hypoglycemia. *J Pediatr.* 2005; **147**(5): 680–5.

Taylor H, Alden J. Age-related differences in outcomes following childhood brain insults: an introduction and overview. *J Int Neuropsychol Soc.* 1997; **3**(6): 555–67.

Vlassara H, Brownlee M, Cerami A. Excessive nonenzymatic glycosylation of peripheral and central nervous system myelin components in diabetic rats. *Diabetes.* 1983; **32**(7): 670–4.

Wysocki T, Harris M, Mauras N, *et al.* Absence of adverse effects of severe hypoglycemia on cognitive function in school-aged children with diabetes over 18 months. *Diabetes Care.* 2003; **26**(4): 1100–5.

Wysocki T, Meinhold P, Cox D, *et al.* Survey of diabetes professionals regarding developmental changes in diabetes self-care. *Diabetes Care.* 1990; **13**(1): 65–8.

Yakovlev PI, Lecours A. The myelogenetic cycles of regional maturation of the brain. In: Minkowski A, editor. *Regional Development of the Brain in Early Life.* Oxford: Blackwell; 1975. pp. 3–64.

Yamada KA, Rensing N, Izumi Y, *et al.* Repetitive hypoglycaemia in young rats impairs hippocampal long-term potentiation. *Pediatr Res.* 2004; **55**(3): 372–9.

CHAPTER 6

Sex, drugs and glycaemic control

Joan-Carles Surís and Christina Akré

INTRODUCTION

Participation in risk (or exploratory) behaviours is part of adolescence, to the point where this can be considered part of normal adolescent development (Michaud *et al.*, 1998; Sawyer *et al.*, 2007). Fortunately, most of these behaviours are very often exploratory and eventually disappear with age (Helgeson *et al.*, 2007; Michaud *et al.*, 1998). There is an emerging literature reporting that chronically ill adolescents engage in risk behaviours as often or even more often than their healthy peers (Sawyer *et al.*, 2007; Surís *et al.*, 2008), and young people with diabetes are no exception (Charron-Prochownik *et al.*, 2006; Kakleas *et al.*, 2009; Scaramuzza *et al.*, 2010). This is worrisome both for parents and for health professionals because these behaviours are associated with poorer adherence to treatment and because young people with diabetes are at increased risk for negative health outcomes (Sawyer *et al.*, 2007). While diabetes complications are extremely rare during adolescence, it is during this period that the progression of risk may accelerate (Daneman, 2005).

Diabetes is a chronic disease implying a lifelong, painful and time-consuming treatment that interferes with daily life and requires self-discipline and a balanced diet. Many adolescents have trouble coping with it (Soltesz, 2009). For young people with diabetes, engaging in risk behaviours may be a way to be accepted by their peers and to prove they are 'normal' (Jack, 2003). Moreover, it may also be a way to deny the condition, albeit temporarily.

The objective of this chapter is to describe the rates of different risk behaviours (smoking, alcohol misuse, use of illegal substances, unsafe sexual practices, sedentary behaviour) among adolescents with diabetes and to consider and respond to the health implications of such behaviours.

EPIDEMIOLOGY OF RISK BEHAVIOURS

There is quite a body of research devoted to adolescents who have diabetes, because it is one of the most frequent chronic conditions. Nevertheless, as for most chronic conditions, epidemiological data on risk behaviours among young people with diabetes have methodological limitations (Sawyer *et al.*, 2007) that need to be taken into account when interpreting data: they are often based on convenience (Falsetti *et al.*, 2003; Martínez-Aguayo, 2007; Scaramuzza *et al.*, 2010) or clinically non-representative samples (Frey *et al.*, 1997; Holl *et al.*, 1998; Hargrave *et al.*, 1999; Michaliszyn *et al.*, 2010; Valerio *et al.*, 2007). They may use non-representative samples or represent different age groups, they may not have a control group (Aman *et al.*, 2009; Amin *et al.*, 2008; Frey *et al.*, 1997; Hofer *et al.*, 2009; Holl *et al.*, 1998; Lièvre *et al.*, 2005; Margeirsdottir *et al.*, 2008; Overby *et al.*, 2009; Schwab *et al.*, 2010), or they may lack standardised measures, both of illness severity and studied behaviours (Lièvre *et al.*, 2005). These limitations will be highlighted as the studies are discussed.

Smoking

Smoking is probably the most studied risk behaviour among adolescents with diabetes because they are at increased risk of vascular disease – a risk that increases if they become smokers. Additionally, smoking may accelerate the progression of microvascular complications (Hargrave *et al.*, 1999; Tyc and Throckmorton-Belzer, 2006). Data comparing smoking rates between

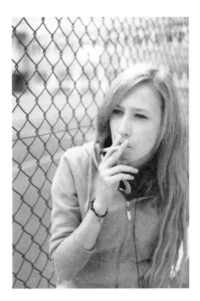

Like all young people, teenagers with diabetes may feel
pressured to do things that are bad for them

adolescents with diabetes and healthy peers are unclear. A Chilean study (Martínez-Aguayo *et al.*, 2007) reported that young people with diabetes were significantly less likely to smoke than controls, while Italian (Scaramuzza *et al.*, 2010) and Swedish (Lodefalk and Aman, 2010) studies found no difference for daily smoking (*see* Table 6.1).

TABLE 6.1 Prevalence of tobacco smoking among young people with diabetes

Author, year (ref)	N	Age group (years)	Group with diabetes	Controls
Frey *et al.*, 1997	155	10–20	34% (ever)	NR
			27% (past 12 months)	
Holl *et al.*, 1998	238	8–29	19.3% (urinary cotinine)	NR
Hargrave *et al.*, 1999	100	6–19	7% (urinary cotinine)	NR
Kyngäs, 2000	289	13–17	11.8% (occasionally)	NR
			35.6% (regularly)	
Lièvre *et al.*, 2005	562	10–16	6.4%	NR
Martínez-Aguayo *et al.*, 2007	193 with diabetes	13–20	60.1% (lifetime prevalence)	75.0%**
			36.2% (annual prevalence)	61.2%**
	58 489 controls		27.7% (30-day prevalence)	37.9%**
Margeirsdottir *et al.*, 2008	1658	1–23	1.5% (girls)	NR
			2.2% (boys)	
Hofer *et al.*, 2009	27 561	0–20	13.7% (daily smoker, girls)	NR
			21.6% (daily smoker, boys)	
Scaramuzza *et al.*, 2010	215 with diabetes	12–18	54.5% (ever, girls)	55.1%
			25.0% (daily, girls)	27.0%
	464 controls		47.4% (ever, boys)	38.1%*
			33.0% (daily, boys)	34.0%
Lodefalk and Aman, 2010	160 with diabetes	13–19	5.6% (daily smokers)	8.2%
	159 controls			
Schwab *et al.*, 2010	33 488	≤ 18	13% (daily smoker, girls)	NR
			15% (daily smoker, boys)	

*p < 0.05; **p < 0.01; NR, not reported.

Young people with diabetes who smoke have worse metabolic control and an increased cardiovascular risk profile compared with non-smokers (Hofer *et al.*, 2009; Jack, 2003; Tyc and Throckmorton-Belzer, 2006). Moreover, among adolescents with diabetes presenting four or five cardiovascular risk factors, 70% were smokers (Schwab *et al.*, 2010). However, a study among 527 young people with diabetes in the United Kingdom found that smoking status was not a predictor of microalbuminuria (Amin *et al.*, 2008), while a French report (Lièvre *et al.*, 2005) indicated that complications were infrequent among adolescents and that smoking did not play a significant role. Others (Martínez-Aguayo *et al.*, 2007) found no difference in HbA$_{1c}$ between smokers and non-smokers.

Alcohol

Alcohol use among young people with diabetes has been associated with a greater degree of glycaemic variation (Ismail *et al.*, 2006), with delayed hypoglycaemia and with an impaired ability to detect hypoglycaemic symptoms (Kakleas *et al.*, 2009). Most studies limit their comparisons to alcohol use (independent of quantity and frequency) between young people with or without diabetes and come up with inconclusive results. For some (Martínez-Aguayo *et al.*, 2007), adolescents with diabetes would report significantly lower rates of lifetime and 30-day prevalence, while for others (Scaramuzza *et al.*, 2010), girls – but not boys – with diabetes show higher rates of alcohol use than controls. Nevertheless, the only study comparing youths having ever been drunk (which is a more accurate indicator of alcohol misuse) found no difference between cases and controls (Scaramuzza *et al.*, 2010) (*see* Table 6.2).

TABLE 6.2 Prevalence of alcohol use and misuse among young people with diabetes

Author, year (ref)	N	Age group (years)	Group with diabetes	Controls
Frey *et al.*, 1997	155	10–20	39% (ever)	NR
			30% (past 12 months)	
Kyngäs, 2000	289	13–17	29.4% (occasionally)	NR
			22.1% (regularly)	
Ismail *et al.*, 2006	14	>16	43% (inebriated)	NR
			14% (to the point of being physically sick)	
Martínez-Aguayo *et al.*, 2007	193 with diabetes	13–20	57.0% (lifetime prevalence)	78.7%**
	58 489 controls		49.5% (annual prevalence)	51.5%
			30.1% (30-day prevalence)	39.2%**
Scaramuzza *et al.*, 2010	215 with diabetes	12–18	65.0% (girls)	51.0%*
	464 controls		56.0% (boys)	61.0%
			87% (girls, ever drunk)	86%
			82% (boys, ever drunk)	83%

*p < 0.05; **p < 0.01; NR, not reported.

CANNABIS AND OTHER ILLEGAL SUBSTANCES

Research on the use of illegal substances among young people with diabetes is scarce and concludes that it may contribute to poor glycaemic control and to serious complications (Kakleas *et al.*, 2009). In the specific case of cannabis, it should be considered as acting like tobacco, because most cannabis users also smoke (Surís *et al.*, 2007), and because cannabis users almost always add tobacco to their cannabis cigarettes (Akré *et al.*, 2010).

Cannabis use also shows divergences in the literature: while a Chilean study (Martínez-Aguayo *et al.*, 2007) reports lower lifetime and annual (but not 30 days) prevalence rates among adolescents with diabetes, an Italian one found higher use rates for females with diabetes and no difference for males (Scaramuzza *et al.*, 2010) (*see* Table 6.3).

TABLE 6.3 Prevalence of cannabis use among young people with diabetes

Author, year (ref)	N	Age group (years)	Group with diabetes	Controls
Frey *et al.*, 1997 (15)	155	10–20	11% (ever)	NR
			8% (past 12 months)	
Martínez-Aguayo *et al.*, 2007 (13)	193 young people with diabetes	13–20	9.6% (lifetime prevalence)	21.7%**
			6.4% (annual prevalence)	12.9%**
	58 489 controls		4.8% (30-day prevalence)	6.7%
Scaramuzza *et al.*, 2010 (6)	215 young people with diabetes	12–18	40.9% (girls)	32.4%*
			38.6% (boys)	38.9%
	464 controls			

*p < 0.05; **p < 0.01; NR, not reported.

Overall, prevalence rates of other illegal substances are low, but they show the same differences as the other studied substances. For some (Martínez-Aguayo *et al.*, 2007) lifetime use rates are higher among controls (but only significant for cocaine and inhalants). For others (Scaramuzza *et al.*, 2010), females with diabetes are significantly more likely to have used illegal drugs other than cannabis, while there are no differences for males (*see* Table 6.4).

It is worth noting that although young people with diabetes may show lower rates of substance use (both legal and illegal) than their healthy counterparts, the difference disappears by grades 11 and 12 (Martínez-Aguayo *et al.*, 2007). This fact could be explained by a delayed pubertal maturation among young people with diabetes (Hsu *et al.*, 2010; Rohrer *et al.*, 2007).

TABLE 6.4 Prevalence of illegal drug use among young people with diabetes

Author, year (ref)	N	Age group (years)	Group with diabetes	Controls
Frey et al., 1997	155	10–20	10% (ever)	NR
			8% (past 12 months)	
Martínez-Aguayo et al., 2007	193 with diabetes 58 489 controls	13–20	1.1% (lifetime cocaine)	5.7%**
			2.7% (lifetime amphetamines)	5.9%
			1.1% (lifetime Ecstasy)	3.3%
			1.6% (lifetime inhalants)	7.9%**
			0.5% (lifetime heroin)	1.4%
Scaramuzza et al., 2010	215 with diabetes 464 controls	12–18	5.0% (girls)	3.0%**
			2.0% (boys)	3.1%

**p $<$ 0.01; NR, not reported.

Unsafe sexual practices

Unsafe sexual practices place female adolescents with diabetes at high risk for unplanned pregnancies and reproductive complications (Charron-Prochownik et al., 2006). The main potential consequences of unintentional pregnancies among women with diabetes are spontaneous abortions and major malformations of newborns (American Diabetes Association, 2004). Other complications such as pre-eclampsia or foetal distress have also been described (Kakleas et al., 2009). This is probably the reason why most research on sexual health among patients with diabetes is limited to females, with little known about condom use in boys. Data including only a small sample of adolescent females show very few differences between girls with diabetes and healthy controls, although the former seem less likely to always use a condom or use protection against unplanned pregnancy (Falsetti et al., 2003). Other studies (Schwarz et al., 2010), also only among girls with diabetes, seem to corroborate these results.

Scaramuzza et al. (2010) report gender differences: while girls with diabetes are significantly less likely to be sexually active than the controls, no differences are observed for boys. This finding could be explained by the fact that the mean age at first intercourse for females with diabetes is almost a year later than for the controls. Moreover, while girls with diabetes are significantly less likely to use contraception than their healthy peers, the reverse is true for males. Charron-Prochownik et al. (2006) showed that male condoms were the main birth control method used by female adolescents with diabetes (94%), followed by the pill (52%) and abstinence (39%). It is worth noting that 38% used no contraception at all and 32% relied on the withdrawal method. No differences were observed with controls (see Table 6.5).

TABLE 6.5 Sexual activity among young people with diabetes

Author, year (ref)	N	Age group (years)	Group with diabetes	Controls
Frey et al., 1997	155	10–20	29% (unprotected intercourse, ever)	NR
Falsetti et al., 2003	37 girls with diabetes 27 controls	16–22	62% (using birth control)	78%
			73% (always using condom)	84%
			78% (protection from unplanned pregnancy)	85%
			70% (protection from sexually transmitted disease)	67%
			11% (history of pregnancy)	7%
			5% (chlamydia infection)	4%
			3% (trichomoniasis infection)	0%
			14% (abnormal pap smear)	15%
Charron-Prochownik et al., 2006	80 girls with diabetes 37 controls	16–20	40% (sexually active)	60%*
			15.7 years (mean age at first intercourse)	16.1 years
			39% (episode of unprotected sex)	48%
			77% (always birth control during sex)	71%
			38% (contraception < 94% effective)	36%
Schwarz et al., 2010	89 girls with diabetes	13–19	24% (sexually active)	NR
			57% (currently using birth control)	
			48% (known risk of unintended pregnancy)	
Scaramuzza et al., 2010	215 young people with diabetes 464 controls	12–18	29% (sexually active, girls)	41%*
			35% (sexually active, boys)	36%
			Mean age at first intercourse	
			17.4 years (girls)	16.5 years
			16.3 years (boys)	15.9 years
			Contraceptive use	
			60% (girls)	79%*
			87% (boys)	70%**

*$p < 0.05$; **$p < 0.01$; NR, not reported.

Physical activity and sedentary behaviours

Physical activity is considered one of the cornerstones in the treatment of diabetes and it is associated with improved insulin sensitivity and lipid profile, as well as with an increased well-being (Aman et al., 2009). In general, patients with diabetes show lower levels of physical activity than their counterparts (Moussa *et al.*, 2005; Valerio *et al.*, 2007). Additionally, they also spend more time on sedentary behaviours than on physical activity (Margeirsdottir *et al.*, 2008; Michaliszyn and Faulkner, 2010; Overby *et al.*, 2009). However, no differences were found regarding compliance with physical activity and electronic media recommendations (Lobelo *et al.*, 2010) (*see* Table 6.6).

TABLE 6.6 Prevalence of physical activity among young people with diabetes

Author, year (ref)	N	Age group (years)	Group with diabetes	Controls
Kyngäs, 2000	289	13–18	42.2% (weekly)	
			51.2% (occasionally)	NR
			6.6% (not at all)	
Moussa *et al.*, 2005	349 with diabetes	6–18	*Physical activity*	
			67.1% (light/very light)	51.6%**
	409 controls		21.9% (moderate)	31.9%
			11.0% (heavy/very heavy)	16.5%
Valerio *et al.*, 2007	138 with diabetes	6–20	*Average days physically active (60 minutes) during last week*	
	269 controls		2.6 (girls)	1.8**
			3.5 (boys)	3.9
			Level of physical activity	
			24.6% (inactive)	7.8%**
			50.7% (moderately active)	55.4%
			24.6% (active)	36.8%
Margeirsdottir *et al.*, 2008	576	1–23	*Sedentary activity > 2 hours/day*	
			99.7% (girls)	NR
			97.7% (boys)	
			Moderate physical activity < 1 hour/day	
			61.1% (girls)	NR
			42.7% (boys)	
Aman *et al.*, 2009	2007	11–18	*Average days physically active (60 minutes) during last week*	
			3.3 (girls)	NR
			4.1 (boys)	

Author, year (ref)	N	Age group (years)	Group with diabetes	Controls
Overby et al., 2009	483	11–19	*Time spent in physical activity (minutes/day, mean)*	
			47 (girls, moderate)	
			3 (girls, vigorous)	NR
			57 (boys, moderate)	
			8 (boys, vigorous)	
			Inactivity (minutes/day, mean)	
			231 (girls)	NR
			263 (boys)	
Michaliszyn and Faulkner, 2010	16	12–17	*Time spent in daily activity*	
			83.5% (sedentary time)	
			10.8% (light activity time)	NR
			5.6% (moderate to vigorous activity time)	
Lobelo et al., 2010	384 with diabetes 173 controls	10–20	*Compliance with recommendations*	
			39% (vigorous activity, girls)	40%
			49% (vigorous activity, boys)	61%
			81% (moderate/vigorous, girls)	77%
			82% (moderate/vigorous, boys)	81%
			49% (electronic media use, girls)	48%
			35% (electronic media use, boys)	35%

**p < 0.01; NR, not reported.

Overall, more than half (54%) of children and adolescents with diabetes do not meet the recommendations for physical activity (Overby et al., 2009). In general, boys are more likely to be physically active than girls (Aman et al., 2009; Overby et al., 2009; Valerio et al., 2007), and physical activity decreases with age (Aman et al., 2009; Overby et al., 2009; Valerio et al., 2007). Interestingly, boys with diabetes are also more likely to spend time on sedentary activities than girls (Aman et al., 2009; Lobelo et al., 2010; Overby et al., 2009). However, the association between physical inactivity and health outcomes is not that clear. Aman et al. (2009) found no association between physical activity and metabolic syndrome, frequency of hypoglycaemia, ketoacidosis or body mass index (BMI). Valerio et al. (2007) found no difference in BMI. Overby et al. (2009) found no association between moderate physical activity and HbA$_{1c}$ when controlling for confounding variables. Other authors (e.g. Michaliszyn and Faulkner, 2010) found that time spent in sedentary activity was associated with increases in cholesterol and triglycerides. Nevertheless, more physically active individuals are less likely to skip meals (Overby *et al.*, 2009) and are more likely to have a positive health perception (Aman *et al.*, 2009).

Clustering of risk behaviours

Adolescents adopting risk behaviours such as smoking, alcohol use and lack of exercise show a lower rate of treatment adherence (Kyngäs, 2000) and management (Scaramuzza *et al.*, 2010; Jack, 2003), and inactive patients with diabetes are more likely to have poorer metabolic control (Valerio *et al.*, 2007). Some studies (Neumark-Sztainer *et al.*, 2002) indicate that both male and female adolescents with diabetes increase their smoking as a way to control their weight. Moreover, daily smokers with diabetes report more gastrointestinal symptoms and have more often irregular meal habits (Lodefalk and Aman, 2010). Young people with diabetes, especially females, have also shown important rates of unhealthy weight control practices (Neumark-Sztainer *et al.*, 2002) (*see* Chapter 13).

NORMAL ADOLESCENT DEVELOPMENT

As already mentioned, exploratory behaviours may be part of normal adolescent development and socialising for young people. In fact, there is some evidence indicating that abstainers are less socially driven and have more trouble with their peers than adolescents using substances (Carter *et al.*, 2007; Hoel *et al.*, 2004; Laukkanen *et al.*, 2001; Tucker *et al.*, 2006; Zambon *et al.*, 2006). It has also been postulated that chronically ill adolescents engage in health-compromising behaviours to prove their 'normality' and to be accepted by their peers (Regber and Kelly, 2007; Surís *et al.*, 2008), although denial of risk could also be another explanation (Regber and Kelly, 2007). From this point of view, even though these behaviours create worry for parents and healthcare teams, engaging in such behaviours may be part of the adolescent's rite of passage.

PREVENTION STRATEGIES

Adolescents with diabetes are frequently in contact with health professionals. Unfortunately, there is evidence indicating that adolescents suffering from chronic conditions such as sickle-cell disease or cystic fibrosis receive preventive counselling only infrequently (Britto *et al.*, 1999; Sawyer *et al.*, 2007; Zack *et al.*, 2003). A qualitative study among young smokers with diabetes (Regber and Kelly, 2007) reported that the diabetes care team was rarely mentioned as a source of information regarding the negative consequences of smoking and that none of the young people who were interviewed mentioned any of the health professionals they had contact with as a resource for helping them to stop. Moreover, over half of all females with diabetes who were aged between 13 and 19 years had not discussed birth control with their healthcare provider, and 70% had no formal instruction on birth control or reported difficulty in accessing it. Additionally, 69% reported not feeling comfortable asking a health professional for birth control (Schwarz et al., 2010). It is also worth mentioning that almost half of health professionals dealing with adolescents with diabetes in the United Kingdom were reported to have received no training in communication skills since graduation and an additional 16% reported they had never received any training (Hambly et al., 2009).

Parents also play an important preventive role in their children's lives, and there is evidence that daughters who have good relationships with their mothers are less likely to engage in risky sexual behaviours (Parera and Surís, 2004). However, this is not always easy. Mothers report problems when having to discuss sexuality issues with their daughters with diabetes. Usually, the trigger for beginning to discuss reproductive health with them is when the daughter has a steady boyfriend. However, mothers also report not being comfortable in engaging in such conversations (Hannan et al., 2009).

WHAT CAN BE DONE?

If we assume that exploratory and/or risky behaviours are part of adolescent development, these issues should be discussed routinely and in a non-threatening way during clinical encounters. A Finnish study (Kyngäs, 2000) indicates that adolescents with diabetes give answers that health professionals want to hear because they believe that they will receive negative responses if they respond truthfully. This also seems to be the case for smokers. Several studies (Hargrave et al., 1999; Holl et al., 1998) report that the number of young people with diabetes who admit to being smokers by questionnaire is lower than when analysing salivary levels of nicotine. Therefore, disclosure of smoking habits would seem to be unreliable (Holl et al., 1998), which suggests that smoking rates among young people with diabetes are probably underestimated. The same is probably true for most health-compromising behaviours. However, prohibiting these behaviours is an ineffective approach, so our efforts should be focused towards harm-reduction strategies (Ismail et al., 2006). The best strategy is probably to give clear, straightforward information about the possible consequences of risk behaviours and to monitor them as closely as possible.

SUMMARY

- Adolescents with diabetes engage in risky behaviours at a similar level to their healthy peers. From this point of view, as reported for other chronic conditions, diabetes is not a protective factor against risk behaviours.
- Most risky behaviours are exploratory and tend to disappear with age. However, longitudinal studies among young people with diabetes are lacking.
- Screening for risk behaviours in a non-threatening way should be part of the routine consultation among young people with diabetes.
- Harm-reduction strategies are probably the best approach in dealing with risk behaviours among young people with diabetes.

REFERENCES

Akré C, Michaud PA, Berchtold A, *et al.* Cannabis and tobacco use: where are the boundaries? A qualitative study on cannabis consumption modes among adolescents. *Health Educ Res.* 2010; **25**(1): 74–82.

Aman J, Skinner TC, de Beaufort CE, *et al.* Associations between physical activity, sedentary behavior, and glycemic control in a large cohort of adolescents with type 1 diabetes: the Hvidoere Study Group on Childhood Diabetes. *Pediatr Diabetes.* 2009; **10**(4): 234–9.

American Diabetes Association. Preconception care of women with diabetes. *Diabetes Care.* 2004; **27**(Suppl. 1): 76–8.

Amin R, Widmer B, Prevost AT, *et al.* Risk of microalbuminuria and progression to macroalbuminuria in a cohort with childhood onset type 1 diabetes: prospective observational study. *BMJ.* 2008; **336**(7646): 697–701.

Britto MT, Garrett JM, Dugliss MA, *et al.* Preventive services received by adolescents with cystic fibrosis and sickle cell disease. *Arch Pediatr Adolesc Med.* 1999; **153**(1): 27–32.

Carter M, McGee R, Taylor B, *et al.* Health outcomes in adolescence: associations with family, friends and school engagement. *J Adolesc.* 2007; **30**(1): 51–62.

Charron-Prochownik D, Sereika SM, Falsetti D, *et al.* Knowledge, attitudes and behaviors related to sexuality and family planning in adolescent women with and without diabetes. *Pediatr Diabetes.* 2006; **7**(5): 267–73.

Daneman D. Early diabetes-related complications in adolescents: risk factors and screening. *Horm Res.* 2005; **63**(2): 75–85.

Falsetti D, Charron-Prochownik D, Serelka S, *et al.* Condom use, pregnancy, and STDs in adolescent females with and without type 1 diabetes. *Diabetes Educ.* 2003; **29**(1): 135–43.

Frey MA, Guthrie B, Loveland-Cherry C, *et al.* Risky behavior and risk in adolescents with IDDM. *J Adolesc Health.* 1997; **20**(1): 38–45.

Hambly H, Robling M, Crowne E, *et al.* Communication skills of healthcare professionals in paediatric diabetes services. *Diabet Med.* 2009; **26**(5): 502–9.

Hannan M, Happ MB, Charron-Prochownik D. Mothers' perspectives about reproductive health discussions with adolescent daughters with diabetes. *Diabetes Educ.* 2009; **35**(2): 265–73.

Hargrave DR, McMaster C, O'Hare MM, *et al.* Tobacco smoke exposure in children and adolescents with diabetes mellitus. *Diabet Med.* 1999; **16**(1): 31–4.

Helgeson VS, Snyder PR, Escobar O, *et al.* Comparison of adolescents with and without diabetes on indices of psychosocial functioning for three years. *J Pediatr Psychol.* 2007; **32**(7): 794–806.

Hoel S, Eriksen BM, Breidablik HJ, *et al.* Adolescent alcohol use, psychological health, and social integration. *Scand J Public Health.* 2004; **32**(5): 361–7.

Hofer SE, Rosenbauer J, Grulich-Henn J, *et al.* Smoking and metabolic control in adolescents with type 1 diabetes. *J Pediatr.* 2009; **154**(1): 20–3.

Holl RW, Grabert M, Heinze E, *et al.* Objective assessment of smoking habits by urinary cotinine measurement in adolescents and young adults with type 1 diabetes: reliability of reported cigarette consumption and relationship to urinary albumin excretion. *Diabetes Care.* 1998; **21**(5): 787–91.

Hsu YY, Dorn LD, Sereika SM. Comparison of puberty and psychosocial adjustment between Taiwanese adolescent females with and without diabetes. *J Clin Nurs.* 2010; **19**(19–20): 2704–12.

Ismail D, Gebert R, Vuillermin PJ, *et al.* Social consumption of alcohol in adolescents with type 1 diabetes is associated with increased glucose lability, but not hypoglycaemia. *Diabet Med.* 2006; **23**(8): 830–3.

Jack L. Biopsychosocial factors affecting metabolic control among female adolescents with type 1 diabetes. *Diabetes Spectrum.* 2003; **16**(3): 154–9.

Kakleas K, Kandyla B, Karayianni C, *et al.* Psychosocial problems in adolescents with type 1 diabetes mellitus. *Diabetes Metab.* 2009; **35**(5): 339–50.

Kyngäs H. Compliance of adolescents with diabetes. *J Pediatr Nurs.* 2000; **15**(4): 260–7.

Laukkanen ER, Shemeikka SL, Viinamaki HT, *et al.* Heavy drinking is associated with more severe psychosocial dysfunction among girls than boys in Finland. *J Adolesc Health.* 2001; **28**(4): 270–7.

Lièvre M, Marre M, Robert JJ, *et al.* Cross-sectional study of care, socio-economic status and complications in young French patients with type 1 diabetes mellitus. *Diabetes Metab.* 2005; **31**(1): 41–6.

Lobelo F, Liese AD, Liu J, *et al.* Physical activity and electronic media use in the SEARCH for diabetes in youth case-control study. *Pediatrics.* 2010; **125**(6): 1364–71.

Lodefalk M, Aman J. Gastrointestinal symptoms in adolescents with type 1 diabetes. *Pediatr Diabetes.* 2010; **11**(4): 265–70.

Margeirsdottir HD, Larsen JR, Brunborg C, *et al.* High prevalence of cardiovascular risk factors in children and adolescents with type 1 diabetes: a population-based study. *Diabetologia.* 2008; **51**(4): 554–61.

Martínez-Aguayo A, Araneda JC, Fernandez D, *et al.* Tobacco, alcohol, and illicit drug use in adolescents with diabetes mellitus. *Pediatr Diabetes.* 2007; **8**(5): 265–71.

Michaliszyn SF, Faulkner MS. Physical activity and sedentary behavior in adolescents with type 1 diabetes. *Res Nurs Health.* 2010; **33**(5): 441–9.

Michaud PA, Blum RW, Ferron C. 'Bet you I will!' Risk or experimental behavior during adolescence? *Arch Pediatr Adolesc Med.* 1998; **152**(3): 224–6.

Moussa MA, Alsaeid M, Abdella N, *et al.* Social and psychological characteristics of Kuwaiti children and adolescents with type 1 diabetes. *Soc Sci Med.* 2005; **60**(8): 1835–44.

Neumark-Sztainer D, Patterson J, Mellin A, *et al.* Weight control practices and disordered eating behaviors among adolescent females and males with type 1 diabetes: associations with sociodemographics, weight concerns, familial factors, and metabolic outcomes. *Diabetes Care.* 2002; **25**(8): 1289–96.

Overby NC, Margeirsdottir HD, Brunborg C, *et al.* Physical activity and overweight in children and adolescents using intensified insulin treatment. *Pediatr Diabetes.* 2009; **10**(2): 135–41.

Parera N, Surís JC. Having a good relationship with their mother: a protective factor against sexual risk behavior among adolescent females? *J Pediatr Adolesc Gynecol.* 2004; **17**(4): 267–71.

Regber S, Kelly KB. Missed opportunities – adolescents with a chronic condition (insulin-dependent diabetes mellitus) describe their cigarette-smoking trajectories and consider health risks. *Acta Paediatr.* 2007; **96**(12): 1770–6.

Rohrer T, Stierkorb E, Heger S, *et al.* Delayed pubertal onset and development in German children and adolescents with type 1 diabetes: cross-sectional analysis of recent data from the DPV diabetes documentation and quality management system. *Eur J Endocrinol.* 2007; **157**(5): 647–53.

Sawyer SM, Drew S, Yeo MS, *et al.* Adolescents with a chronic condition: challenges living, challenges treating. *Lancet.* 2007; **369**(9571): 1481–9.

Scaramuzza A, De Palma A, Mameli C, *et al.* Adolescents with type 1 diabetes and risky behaviour. *Acta Paediatr.* 2010; **99**(8): 1237–41.

Schwab KO, Doerfer J, Marg W, *et al.* Characterization of 33 488 children and adolescents with type 1 diabetes based on the gender-specific increase of cardiovascular risk factors. *Pediatr Diabetes.* 2010; **11**(5): 357–63.

Schwarz EB, Sobota M, Charron-Prochownik D. Perceived access to contraception among adolescents with diabetes: barriers to preventing pregnancy complications. *Diabetes Educ.* 2010; **36**(3): 489–94.

Soltesz G. Worldwide childhood type 1 diabetes epidemiology. *Endocrinol Nutr.* 2009; **56**(Suppl. 4): 53–5.

Surís JC, Akré C, Berchtold A, *et al.* Some go without a cigarette: characteristics of cannabis users who have never smoked tobacco. *Arch Pediatr Adolesc Med.* 2007; **161**(11): 1042–7.

Surís JC, Michaud PA, Akré C, *et al.* Health risk behaviors in adolescents with chronic conditions. *Pediatrics.* 2008; **122**(5): e1113–e1118.

Tucker JS, Ellickson PL, Collins RL, *et al.* Are drug experimenters better adjusted than abstainers and users?: a longitudinal study of adolescent marijuana use. *J Adolesc Health.* 2006; **39**(4): 488–94.

Tyc VL, Throckmorton-Belzer L. Smoking rates and the state of smoking interventions for children and adolescents with chronic illness. *Pediatrics.* 2006; **118**(2): e471–e487.

Valerio G, Spagnuolo MI, Lombardi F, *et al.* Physical activity and sports participation in children and adolescents with type 1 diabetes mellitus. *Nutr Metab Cardiovasc Dis.* 2007; **17**(5): 376–82.

Zack J, Jacobs CP, Keenan PM, *et al.* Perspectives of patients with cystic fibrosis on preventive counseling and transition to adult care. *Pediatr Pulmonol.* 2003; **36**(5): 376–83.

Zambon A, Lemma P, Borraccino A, *et al.* Socio-economic position and adolescents' health in Italy: the role of the quality of social relations. *Eur J Public Health.* 2006; **16**(6): 627–32.

PART II

Management and Intervention

Integrated care and multidisciplinary teamwork: the role of the different professionals

Rebecca Thompson, Alan Delamater,
Rebecca Gebert and Deborah Christie

INTRODUCTION

There is an international consensus about the care of children and young people with diabetes being provided by multidisciplinary teams. It is clearly established that the best model of care for children and young people has at its centre a well-resourced multidisciplinary team (Williamson, 2010). International evidence-based guidelines for the management of children and adolescents with type 1 diabetes published in the last decade strongly support the need for multidisciplinary approaches for the care and management of diabetes (*see* Box 7.1). Following international guidelines, several countries have also expanded and complemented the guidelines with local policies (*see* Box 7.2 for an example).

The recommendations regarding team composition and roles vary slightly. Nevertheless, there is an overall consensus that safe and effective diabetes care demands a multidisciplinary team offering integrated care. Those guidelines emphasise that individuals in the team should include members with appropriate training and competencies in clinical, educational, dietetic, lifestyle, mental health and foot care aspects of diabetes for children and young people. There is acknowledgement that team composition may have geographical variance among countries and within regions, depending on how services are commissioned (e.g. locally or regionally). It may be the case that services provided in low population density areas do not allow for this multidisciplinary structure being feasible. One suggestion is that the expertise should be available via a diabetes care team in regional centres of excellence. An example of the lack of availability of specialist services was reflected in a national UK survey, Minding the Gap (Diabetes UK, 2008). It was found that 85% of people with diabetes in the United Kingdom have either no defined access to psychological support and care or, at best, access to a local generic mental health service only. Less than 3% of diabetes services meet all six psychologically relevant UK National Institute for Health and Clinical Excellence[1] recommendations and National Service Framework[2] standards, and 26% do not meet any. At the time of writing, only 20% of children and adolescent services in the United Kingdom have adequate access to psychological services.

This chapter considers the individual and overlapping roles of the different members of the multidisciplinary team and discusses the essential philosophy required in order for the multidisciplinary team to be truly effective.

BOX 7.1 International guidelines

- Clinical Practice Consensus Guidelines.
- International Society for Pediatric and Adolescent Diabetes (ISPAD) Clinical Practice Consensus Guidelines (2009).
- Type 1 diabetes: diagnosis and management of type 1 diabetes in children and young people. Clinical guidelines, National Institute for Clinical Excellence, United Kingdom (NICE, 2004).
- Care of Children and Adolescents with type 1 diabetes: a statement of the American Diabetes Association (Silverstein *et al.*, 2005).
- Clinical Practice Guidelines for the prevention and management of diabetes in Canada, Canadian Diabetes Association (CDA, 2008).
- Clinical Practice Guidelines: type 1 diabetes in children and adolescents, National Diabetes Strategy Group, Australian Paediatric Endocrine Group (APEG, 2005).

---

1 NICE: an independent organisation responsible for providing national guidance on promoting good health and preventing ill health.
2 NSF: sets strategies that set quality requirements for care based upon available evidence.

BOX 7.2 Specific policies in the United Kingdom

Department of Health
- National Service Framework for Diabetes
- National Service Framework for Diabetes: standards (DoH, 2001)
- National Service Framework for Diabetes: delivery strategy (DoH, 2002)
- Making Every Young Person with Diabetes Matter (DoH, 2007)
- Report of the Children and Young People with Diabetes Working Group (DoH, 2007)

National Institute for Health and Clinical Excellence
- Type 1 Diabetes: diagnosis and management of type 1 diabetes in children and young people; NICE clinical guideline 15 (NICE, 2004)

Royal College of Nursing
- Children and Young people with diabetes: RCN guidance for newly-appointed nurse specialists (RCN 2011)
- Specialist Nursing Services for Children and Young People with Diabetes (RCN, 2006)

Diabetes UK
- When Your Child Has Diabetes: what care to expect (Diabetes UK, 2008)

THE MULTIDISCIPLINARY TEAM

An effective team requires leadership and vision. In the majority of teams, the consultant paediatrician, who should have a special knowledge and/or interest in diabetes, occupies this position. It is increasingly recognised that a basic training in endocrinology is insufficient to offer a safe and effective diabetes service, and there is a need for specialist diabetes education and training.

In services without a multidisciplinary team, a referral to a different department (e.g. a mental health team or a dietetics service) may be made; however, when healthcare providers work independently, there is often no consistent or better understanding gained by their additional involvement. This means that the cycle of assessment, review and referral continues until everyone in the multidisciplinary team, and more, have been involved, with no improvement in glycaemic control.

This can have a significant impact on the child or adolescent and their family, who may have developed further diabetes-related stress, poor self-esteem and feelings of hopelessness that have all been reinforced by being referred from one person to another, resulting in increasing non-attendance rates. This vicious cycle creates a story of failure on the part of the family ('I cannot be fixed') and a view that 'the responsibility for fixing them . . . lies . . . with the physician, the nurse, or the overall health care system' (Rollnick et al, 2008, p. 4). This approach does not explore the 'real' issue for the child or adolescent and their family – what do they need to know about living with diabetes and their health behaviours to support the treatment process? Do they need to clarify and renegotiate the treatment approach to allow their health-seeking behaviours to improve, change or just be supported?

In a multidisciplinary team, various members of the team in addition to the paediatrician should routinely assess diabetes management skills, including knowledge and problem-solving, goals, adherence and self-care autonomy. As they become older, many children are given self-care autonomy without sufficient cognitive and emotional maturity. Interventions that appropriately involve parents are essential, as research has shown that regimen adherence problems are common in older children and adolescents. Parental involvement in children's diabetes care should be evaluated routinely, and interventions delivered to promote teamwork so that good regimen adherence and control of diabetes can be achieved. There is empirical support for these approaches, as a number of controlled studies have shown that interventions to improve parent–adolescent teamwork in diabetes management resulted in less conflict and better adherence (Ryden *et al.*, 1994; Wysocki *et al.*, 2006; Ellis *et al.*, 2005).

BOX 7.3 Members of the multidisciplinary team (MDT)

As a minimum, the team should consist of the following professionals:

- A *consultant paediatrician* with a special knowledge and/or interest in diabetes, who will take overall responsibility for the child or young person's diabetes care and work with the other members of the team.
- A *diabetes nurse specialist* or *diabetes nurse educator* who can give advice and support for managing diabetes in hospital, at home, at school and in other settings.
- A *dietitian* or *nutritionist* who can give advice and support on the family's food to ensure good diabetes control and healthy growth.
- A *clinical psychologist* or access to a *psychological therapies professional* who is, where possible, an integrated member of the team, with experience in diabetes and who can offer support for emotional distress or difficulties connected with living with diabetes.

The MDT may enlist other professionals for patients to have:

- Access to school and social support.
- Access to specialised services, such as ophthalmology and podiatry.

ROLES OF THE DIFFERENT PROFESSIONALS

Paediatrician

The primary role of the paediatrician is to take overall responsibility for delivery of the diabetes care. The paediatrician will take a lead in making decisions about initial investigations at the time of diagnosis, as well as working with the diabetes nurse, the child or young person and their family to make decisions about the most acceptable and appropriate regimen. The paediatrician usually has responsibility for reviewing the impact of the treatment regimen and prescribing changes to the frequency and amount of insulin to be injected or delivered via a pump. In the United Kingdom, some nurses are gaining a qualification in prescribing, and in some other countries different health professionals may also prescribe, so they may be able to undertake this role as well as the paediatrician.

Research has demonstrated that children who have infrequent and irregular contact with the healthcare team are more likely to have significant problems with metabolic control (Kaufman *et al.*, 1999; Jacobson *et al.*, 1997). However, the frequency of contact with families can differ dramatically, ranging from monthly to 6-monthly. In many clinics, the paediatrician's role is to review the blood glucose records and glycaemic control (HbA1c). If these are felt to be 'unsatisfactory', it is likely that actions to solve the problem/s and to improve the glycaemic control will be agreed (Brink *et al.*, 2002). If there is no significant improvement in glycaemic control at the next clinic visit, the most likely outcome will be referral to another member of the team.

Nurse specialist

A diabetes nurse specialist or diabetes nurse educator is the second essential member of a diabetes team. In the United Kingdom, the diabetes nurse specialist is an experienced children's nurse with additional diabetes-related theoretical and practical knowledge, as well as management experience at ward level or equivalent. Nurses working in these roles are expected to develop further professionally undertaking a master's or PhD. In several countries outside the United Kingdom, the role of diabetes educator has been developed. This role is described in detail in Chapter 10.

The nurse may be based either in hospital or within the community, and this may influence both the responsibilities that the individual holds and where they are able to see a child and their family. An overview of the nursing role can be described under the following subheadings.

The role of the diabetes nurse specialist

The Royal College of Nursing (RCN, 2006) describes three levels of role development for nurses working within paediatric diabetes care.

1. *Diabetes specialist nurse*: this is the entry point where the individual would be considered an 'advanced beginner' and becomes 'proficient'.
2. *Clinical nurse specialist*: the individual starts as 'proficient', with the aim of developing to function at 'expert' level.
3. *Nurse consultant*: where the individual functions at expert level.

Clinical expert

The Royal College of Nursing (RCN, 2004) describes how the paediatric diabetes specialist nurse is likely to be the core of the multidisciplinary team. The nurse specialist is the person who coordinates with other healthcare professionals, assessing, planning and evaluating programs of care. They are likely to be the first port of call to assist children, young people and their families and the source of expert advice, via telephone or face-to-face consultations. This includes insulin dose management for glucose levels, food, illness and exercise.

Educator

In the United Kingdom, the majority of education is delivered by diabetes specialist nurses, with differing levels of support from other members of the diabetes team. Education will be provided in a variety of environments, including hospital, outpatient clinics, schools and homes and it may be informal, on a one-to-one basis, or more structured, in groups covering specific topics.

Nurse specialists will meet the child and family at diagnosis, providing the initial skills teaching to ensure that they are safe to manage in their own home. They will provide ongoing assessment of the child or young person's adjustment to diabetes, facilitating age-appropriate transfer of knowledge and care to the adolescent when appropriate. The paediatric nurse specialist will also liaise and provide support and expert advice to other key members who support the child, including parents, carers, ward staff and staff at school, such as teachers and school nurses. The nurse specialist is also a technical expert and will be able to provide education on blood glucose and ketone meters, insulin pens and insulin pumps.

Advocate

The nurse specialist is often the constant member of the diabetes team and the team member who is most likely to see the family on a regular basis. As a consequence, they are available to provide support for children, young people and families, helping them navigate their diabetes journey. They are often the individuals who are able to identify the barriers to successful diabetes control, such as fear of hypoglycaemia (*see* Chapter 3) and the young person's sense of being different from his or her peers (*see* Chapters 2, 6 and 14).

Dietitian/nutritionist

As indicated by the nutritional management Clinical Practice Consensus Guidelines (ISPAD, 2009), nutritional management is one of the cornerstones of diabetes care and education. A paediatric dietitian is a key member of the multidisciplinary diabetes team.

A paediatric dietitian will have a minimum of 2 years' postgraduate experience prior to specialising in paediatrics, as well as a specific qualification in paediatric dietetics. They would be expected to have completed or to be working towards a master's level qualification, with training in paediatric diabetes and medicines management.

The paediatric dietitian provides information and training on how glycaemic control is influenced by routines in relation to meal and snack times and can discuss fluctuations in appetite caused by growth velocity and how to achieve a balance between insulin action, food intake and energy expenditure. They can provide advice on:

- bolus choices with meals relating to glycaemic index and fat and protein content
- manipulation of diet for weight management and exercise/sports nutrition advice
- managing coeliac disease and cystic fibrosis
- diabetes-related conditions that have other nutritional implications (renal disease, oncology patients with specific nutritional needs, enteral feeds).

The International Society of Pediatric and Adolescent Diabetes (ISPAD) recommends a minimum contact with the dietitian should include two to four meetings in the first year following diagnosis, with an annual reassessment for review and education. Contact should be more frequent when a child develops coeliac disease or dyslipidaemia and when insulin regimens are reviewed.

Psychologist

A substantial research base has established the significant role of psychosocial factors in paediatric diabetes management. The ISPAD recently published guidelines for the psychological care of young people with diabetes (Delamater, 2009). The guidelines state that the interdisciplinary healthcare team should include mental health or behavioural health professionals who can screen and assess psychosocial functioning, both generally and specifically in relation to diabetes management tasks. Research has shown that young people who do not manage diabetes well and who have poor glycaemic control are more likely to have more family conflict and less parent involvement and support for diabetes tasks. They are also more likely to experience psychological problems, such as depression and eating disorders. These considerations suggest that psychosocial factors should be routinely assessed, preferably by a psychologist who is also knowledgeable about diabetes and its management. (As an adjunct to this, there should be access to psychiatric assessment in cases of severe psychopathology that may compromise diabetes management.[3]) Another important function of the psychologist is to assess developmental progress in all domains of life, including psychological, social and academic, and diabetes-specific functioning.

The traditional consultation model, where individuals' needs are identified and referrals are made to another professional who is then able to 'consult' the psychologist about intervention, is less likely to be as effective as having the psychologist function as part of the healthcare team. When referrals to outside teams are made for evaluation and treatment, many people do not follow through on referrals – especially if they are at a different location and time. Another advantage to having a psychologist as part of the team is the potential for training other members in the identification of problem behaviours, as well as simple counselling techniques that may improve patient adherence, and how and when to refer to the psychologist. This is desirable, since it is unlikely that the psychologist or other mental health professional could possibly see all people coming to clinic appointments (*see* Chapter 12).

Other professionals/services involved
Chiropodist/podiatrist
Chiropodists (or podiatrists) assess, diagnose and treat abnormalities and diseases of the lower limb. The microvascular changes caused by poor diabetes control mean that specialist care for foot ailments, ranging from problems such as verrucas, warts and fungal skin and nail infections, is essential. A chiropodist/podiatrist can also give professional advice on the prevention of foot problems, raise awareness and give advice about footwear or foot health. Issues specific to children include hypermobility, which can cause pain in the knees, hips or feet. To try to alleviate these problems, insoles can be used to help with the biomechanics of the foot. Young children, particularly boys who are keen

---

3　NHS Diabetes (2011) *Emotional and Psychological Support and Care in Diabetes.* Newcastle upon Tyne: NHS Diabetes.

on sport, can experience Sever's disease heel pain as the calcaneum and joint spaces are maturing. Again, insoles can help with this problem.

Ophthalmologist

An ophthalmologist provides the medical and surgical management of conditions in and around the eye. The most important impact of diabetes on the eye is diabetic retinopathy, which is responsible for most of the sight-threatening complications of diabetes. Retinopathy is the most common complication of diabetes; up to 10% of people living with diabetes at any one time will have sight-threatening retinopathy requiring specialist ophthalmological management (Negi and Vernon, 2003). With adolescents having a higher risk of progression to vision-threatening retinopathy than adults (ISPAD, 2009), it is important to refer this age group for screening.

School nurse

In the United Kingdom, school nurses can be employed by the local health authority, primary care trust or community trust or by the school directly. State sector school nurses cover an average of 7.5 schools – one secondary school and six primary schools, which equates to 2590 pupils. Independent school nurses typically only provide a service in one school, covering an average of 663 pupils (Ball, 2009). A school nurse is a registered nurse who has successfully completed a post-registration graduate programme and is registered as a 'specialist community public health practitioner' (school nurse).[4] School nurses provide a variety of services that may include providing education, carrying out developmental screening, undertaking health interviews, attending child protection conferences and administering immunisation programmes. The school nurse is ideally placed to support a child or adolescent living with diabetes while they are in school; for example, they can help with supervising injections at lunchtime and supporting the treatment of hypo- and hyperglycaemia. However, one state sector school nurse covers an average of 7.5 schools (typically one secondary school and six primary schools), equating to an average total of 2590 pupils (Ball 2009). This makes it virtually impossible for the school nurse to be involved in the day-to-day management of diabetes. However, school nurses can be helpful members of the multidisciplinary team when thinking about supporting training of school staff, completion of school medical management plans and facilitating the link between schools/pupils and the diabetes team.

---

4   Department of Health (2006) *School Nurse: practice development resource pack.* London: DoH.

WORKING AS A TEAM

Although there is general consensus among the diabetes community about involvement of a multidisciplinary diabetes healthcare team, there still remains little consensus about the underlying approach of teams towards childhood diabetes (Drotar *et al.*, 2010). If the primary goal of the team is to improve its understanding of children and adolescents, allow them to make choices to integrate diabetes into their lives and support intensive diabetes self-management, an 'individualised' healthcare approach needs to be adopted (Brink and Moltz, 1997). This means it is essential to find ways to understand the challenges faced by each child, adolescent and family.

Skinner and Cameron (2010, p. 373) argue that 'it is essential for a team to consider childhood differences with an aim to appreciate individual ability to achieve optimal health outcomes', and that a 'one size fits all approach' does not accommodate children, adolescents with diabetes or their families.

A sense of harmony within the team enables a consistent approach to help create trust between the family and the healthcare professionals. Brink and colleagues (2002) argue that teams that value the cohesive, shared understanding and collaborative practice (evidenced in documentation, communication and meetings) deliver care that enhances 'patient . . . and . . . family's fund of knowledge' (p. 3). Adopting this approach means that everyone complements or adds their specialty to the experience for the family. Each team member understands their role and their value in the team.

Team members need to embrace a shared communication style that invites children, young people and their families to work as part of a collaborative team. This means avoiding oppositional language such as 'good' or 'bad', as well as avoiding language that implies value judgements and blame. Collaboration among the team in information collection through team and family discussions can document points of view, beliefs and understanding collected from the child, or their family. It can also prevent repetition in consultations with different team members and foster a sense of seamless interaction with the family (Brink *et al.*, 2002).

SUMMARY

Local and international guidelines emphasise the importance of a multidisciplinary team approach to manage diabetes in children and young people. Common sense indicates that an effective multidisciplinary team needs much more than just a collection of different individuals with different training and qualifications: the individuals must be working and cooperating together, as this will have a considerable impact on patient and diabetes management.

REFERENCES

Australasian Paediatric Endocrine Group (APEG). *Clinical Practice Guidelines: type 1 diabetes in children and adolescents.* Canberra: National Health and Medical Research Council; 2005. Available at: www.nhmrc.gov.au/guidelines/publications/cp102%20 (accessed 18 December 2011).

Ball J. *School Nursing in 2009: Results from a survey of RCN members working in schools in 2009.* Royal College of Nursing (RCN) & Employment Research; 2009.

Brink SJ, Miller M, Moltz KC. Education and multidisciplinary team care concepts for pediatric and adolescent diabetes mellitus. *J Pediatr Endocrinol Metab.* 2002; **15**(8): 1113–30.

Brink SJ, Moltz K. The message of the DCCT for children and adolescents. *Diabetes Spectrum.* 1997; **10**(4): 259–67.

Canadian Diabetes Association (CDA). Clinical Practice Guidelines. *Can J Diabetes.* 2008 **32**(Suppl 1): 1–215.

Delamater AM. Psychological care of children and adolescents with diabetes. *Pediatr Diabetes.* 2009; **10**(Suppl. 12): 175–84.

Department of Health (DoH). *National Service Framework for Diabetes: standards.* 2001. London: DoH.

Department of Health (DoH). *National Service Framework for Diabetes: delivery strategy.* 2002. London: DoH.

Department of Health (DoH). *Making Every Young Person with Diabetes Matter: report of the children and young people with diabetes working group.* DoH; 2007. London: DoH.

Diabetes UK. *Minding the Gap: the provision of psychological support and care.* Diabetes UK; 2008a. Available at: www.diabetes.org.uk/Documents/Reports/Minding_the_Gap_psychological_report.pdf (accessed 18 December 2011).

Diabetes UK. *When Your Child Has Diabetes: what care to expect.* Diabetes UK; 2008b. Available at: www.diabetes.org.uk/upload/When%20child%20has%20diabetes.pdf (accessed 18 December 2011).

Drotar D, Crawford P, Bonner M. Collaborative decision-making and promoting treatment adherence in pediatric chronic illness. *Patient Intelligence.* 2010; **2**: 1–7.

Ellis DA, Naar-King S, Frey M, *et al.* Multisystemic treatment of poorly controlled type 1 diabetes: effects on medical resource utilization. *J Pediatr Psychol.* 2005; **30**(8): 656–66.

International Society for Pediatric and Adolescent Diabetes (ISPAD). ISPAD Clinical Practice Consensus Guidelines. *Pediatr Diabetes.* 2009; **10**(Suppl. 12): 1–210.

Jacobson AM, Hauser ST, Willett J, *et al.* Consequences of irregular versus continuous medical follow-up in children and adolescents with insulin-dependent diabetes mellitus. *J Pediatrics.* 1997; **131**(5): 727–33.

Kaufman FR, Halvorson M, Carpenter S. Association between diabetes control and visits to a multidisciplinary pediatric clinic. *Pediatrics.* 1999; **103**(5 Pt. 1): 948–51.

National Institute for Clinical Excellence (NICE). *Type 1 Diabetes: diagnosis and management of type 1 diabetes in children, young people and adults: NICE clinical guideline 15.* London: NICE; 2004.

Negi A, Vernon SA. An overview of the eye in diabetes. *J R Soc Med.* 2003; **96**(6): 266–72.

Royal College of Nursing (RCN). *Children and Young People with Diabetes: RCN guidance for newly-appointed nurse specialists.* Available at: www.rcn.org.uk/__data/assets/pdf_file/0009/78633/002474.pdf (accessed 18 December 2011).

Royal College of Nursing (RCN). *Specialist Nursing Services for Children and Young People with Diabetes.* RCN; 2006. Available at: www.rcn.org.uk/__data/assets/pdf_file/0009/78687/003015.pdf (accessed 18 December 2011).

Ryden L, Nevander P, Johnsson K, *et al.* Family therapy in poorly controlled juvenile IDDM: effects on diabetic control, self-evaluation and behavioural symptoms. *Acta Paediatr.* 1994; **83**(3): 285–91.

Silverstein J, Klingensmith G, Copeland K, *et al.* Care of children and adolescents with type 1 diabetes: a statement of the American Diabetes Association. *Diabetes Care.* 2005: **28**(1): 186–212.

Skinner TC, Cameron FJ. Improving glycaemic control in children and adolescents: which aspects of therapy really matter? *Diabet Med.* 2010; **27**(4): 369–75.

Williamson S. The best model of care for children and young people with diabetes. *J R Coll Physicians Edinb.* 2010; **40**(Suppl. 17): 25–32.

Wysocki T, Harris M, Buckloh L, *et al.* Effects of behavioral family systems therapy for diabetes on adolescents' family relationships, treatment adherence, and metabolic control. *J Pediatr Psychol.* 2006; **31**(9): 928–38.

CHAPTER 8

An introduction to managing diabetes: implications of different treatment regimens

Russell Viner

INTRODUCTION

As highlighted in the earlier chapters, the goals of diabetes management are essentially those of adequate control of blood glucose (glycaemic control) while maintaining a high quality of life. Of course, a great deal hinges on the definition of 'adequate' glycaemic control. Until the late 1980s, it was widely assumed that for children, adequate control meant simply the avoidance of the extremes of hypo- or hyperglycaemia. Better control of blood glucose was thought to be mainly a concern in adults, in order to prevent long-term vascular complications. A series of studies from the 1990s onwards have made it clear that tight glycaemic control is important to attain and maintain from the point of diagnosis, whatever the age (White *et al.*, 2001).

Modern diabetes regimens aim to normalise blood glucose through attempting to mimic normal healthy insulin-glucose physiology. Each new advance in insulin, such as the development of ultra-short-acting analogue insulin, or such devices as insulin pumps and continuous glucose monitors, opens up the possibility of more closely mimicking normal physiology. Better mimicry of normal glucose physiology potentially provides better glycaemic control, thus preventing hypo- and hyperglycaemia and reducing long-term complications (*see* Chapter 1).

Figure 8.1 shows the normal pattern of physiological insulin secretion in those without diabetes, together with insulin levels achieved by multiple daily injections and an insulin pump.

Panel A: Physiological insulin secretion

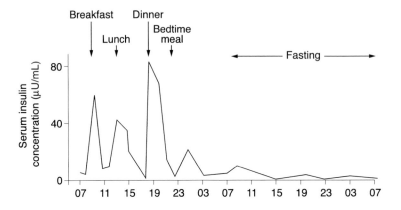

Panel B: Insulin levels with injection regimes

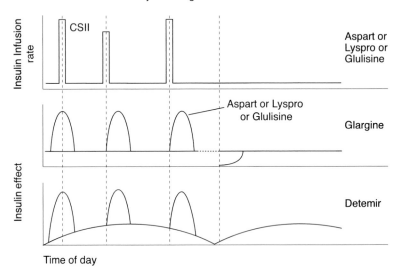

Panel C: Insulin levels with insulin pump theory

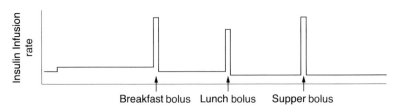

FIGURE 8.1 Normal pattern of physiological insulin secretion

Sources: A, www.harmelphoto.com/KnolType1/seruminsulin.png
        B, www.deo.ucsf.edu/images/graphs/graph_intense_type2.gif
        C, www.deo.ucsf.edu/images/graphs/graph_pump_regimen.gif

As shown in Figure 8.1, we are achieving ever better mimicry of physiological glucose control with more intensive regimens. However, the tantalising goal of the best levels of glycaemic control requires a correspondingly high level of input from young people and their families. Modern diabetes regimens can be very demanding, placing a large daily burden on young people and their family. This burden is repeated daily across the long years of their life. Attaining good diabetes control on a single day is a great achievement, but one that inevitably requires the need to do it all over again the following day – and the next. And the next. Few individuals without diabetes can understand how oppressive modern diabetes regimens can be for young people. It can be argued that this lack of understanding includes the vast majority of healthcare professionals managing diabetes in the young.

In this chapter, we will revisit the practicalities that young people with diabetes have to face in their everyday living. We will follow the young person's advocate perspective to bring a different perspective to this problem.

A DAY IN THE LIFE OF A YOUNG PERSON WITH DIABETES

Let us think through a day in the life of a young person with diabetes who is working hard to achieve good control. For most of us, the day starts with an alarm, perhaps a hurried shower or breakfast, then the trip to school or work. For a young person with diabetes, life is very different. The alarm is quickly followed by:
- a finger prick and blood glucose test
- a calculation of the insulin dose needed for the carbohydrate in the breakfast they are planning
- a consideration of whether a correction dose of insulin needs to be added to the meal insulin
- an injection or pump bolus of insulin (having entered the breakfast carbohydrates and blood glucose value into the pump to allow it to calculate the dose)
- breakfast itself – in an ideal world, breakfast should be a nutritious balanced meal with only long-acting carbohydrates
- the young person on multiple daily injections may also have a dose of long-acting insulin in the morning as well.

The difference between the young person with diabetes and their healthy counterpart without diabetes has started – and it's only 7 a.m.!

Moving on in the morning, for most young people the trip to school requires little thought, simply jumping in the waiting car, running to the bus or, best of all, walking to school. For our young person with diabetes, even the simple trip to school requires some thought:

- Do they have glucose available in their school bag, in case of hypoglycaemia?
- Do they have an insulin pen in their school bag?
- If they're walking to school, is there a risk of hypoglycaemia?
- If so, should they have some carbohydrate or check the blood glucose again on the way?

Once at school, morning break arrives after a couple of hours of lessons. For healthy young people, the morning break is an opportunity to have a snack, chat with friends and possibly play a brief game or kick a ball with friends. For our young person with diabetes, any snacks should be accompanied by a blood glucose check, thought about whether insulin is needed to cover the carbohydrate in the snack (which they will have had to count) and a potential injection or pump bolus. Any activity, games or fun with friends needs to be thought about in relation to the possibility of hypoglycaemia.

It's only 11 a.m., but already our young person with diabetes has potentially needed to think about diabetes or take action 12 or 13 times in a routine day. If things have been more difficult, e.g. they've had an unexpected hypoglycaemic event during a morning lesson and needed to treat it, this could be considerably more.

Figure 8.2 outlines a day in the life of a young person trying hard to achieve good control on injections or a pump. The rest of the day for young people with diabetes repeats much of the work of the morning, thinking about testing, injections and diet with each meal or snack and worrying about hypos with any activity. For many young people who play sport after school, diabetes again looms large. Healthy young people simply throw themselves into the fun. Those with diabetes need to think about blood glucose testing before and potentially during exercise, additional carbohydrate (counted and calculated) if needed, plus potential temporary modifications to basal rates for pump users. Bedtime requires more work. While healthy young people simply fall asleep, those with diabetes need to check their blood glucose before bed and potentially have a snack to avoid overnight hypoglycaemia. Young people on multiple daily doses may need to take their final long-acting insulin.

Figure 8.2 shows that a routine day in which diabetes is well controlled may need up to 35 separate diabetes-related 'adherence points' at which thoughts or actions related to diabetes are needed. Any unpredictable high or low blood glucose results on the way may require further work, as may illness, unaccustomed exercise (e.g. a sports day) or an unaccustomed meal or night out (e.g. a festival or party).

Time	Event	Considerations	Blood glucose	Carb counting and dose calculation	Insulin	Food: diabetic diet
6 a.m.						
7 a.m.	Alarm		✓	✓	✓	✓
8 a.m.	Trip to school	Prepare for school				
9 a.m.						
10 a.m.						
11 a.m.	Break	Exercise?	✓	✓	✓	✓
12 noon						
1 p.m.	Lunch	Exercise	✓	✓	✓	✓
2 p.m.						
3 p.m.	After school	Exercise – sports or walking home	✓			✓
4 p.m.	Snack		✓	✓	✓	✓
5 p.m.						
6 p.m.	Dinner		✓	✓	✓	✓
7 p.m.						
8 p.m.						
9 p.m.	Snack		✓	✓	✓	✓
10 p.m.	Bedtime		✓		✓	
11 p.m.						
12 midnight						

FIGURE 8.2 Daily routine for a young person on multiple daily injections

THE BALANCE BETWEEN CONTROL OF DIABETES AND CONTROL OF LIFE

This level of adherence (*see* Chapter 4) has the potential to dramatically impact on quality of life for young people and their families. While other chronic conditions in children and adolescents may be more visible, more disabling, have greater daily symptoms and be more life-threatening, no other chronic condition is as oppressive as diabetes in the constancy of its demands. As our diabetes regimens become more 'physiological', so too does the requirement for more constant self-surveillance and adherence. We, as health professionals, contribute to this by constantly redefining what 'appropriate' diabetes control is.

In the second decade of the twenty-first century, we continue to constantly redefine good control. HbA$_{1c}$ targets for children and adolescents become increasingly ambitious and regimens become increasingly demanding. What we learn from pumps we then take back into multiple daily injection regimens. In the mid-1990s, many argued that the new gold-standard regimen for children and adolescents was the so-called basal bolus regimen of four injections per day, one long-acting and three meal-related doses, with all doses prescribed by health professionals. Some disagreed, noting there was little evidence that multiple injection regimens improved HbA$_{1c}$ in children, and many children continued to be managed on twice-daily mixed insulin regimens (Betts *et al.*, 2002). However, at the time of writing, the gold-standard regimen of the 1990s now looks like a dinosaur. Even for those not on a pump, the gold standard consists of carbohydrate counting and adjusting insulin dose for carbohydrates with each meal and any snacks using a personal insulin-to-carbohydrates ratio, together with more intense monitoring and correction of hyperglycaemia using personal insulin-sensitivity ratios. As health professionals gain experience with such regimens, we are more confident to suggest correcting ever-lower levels of hyperglycaemia. There is an increasing view that argues that blood glucose over 8 should be corrected, rather than blood glucose over 14 mmol/L. Given recent evidence, these trends towards intensification are likely to continue (Gosden *et al.*, 2010).

Therefore, there is an uneasy tension between 'adequate' glycaemic control and 'acceptable' quality of life. Better health demands constant surveillance, thought and action. However, the stresses of constant surveillance and diabetes-related adherence points mark young people out as different to their peers, intrude on other activities and prevent them living 'normal' lives. This is not a simple spectrum between quality of life at one end and good diabetes control on the other. Modern intensive regimens may improve well-being, through allowing greater flexibility in eating and exercise and through the immediate benefits of better blood glucose control on energy levels, well-being and general health. Many young people, especially those in their teens, achieve reasonable HbA$_{1c}$ levels consistently, despite using non-intensive regimens (e.g. twice-daily injections), without apparently suffering excessive hypoglycaemia.

Health professionals frequently fail to recognise that the uneasy balance between control and quality of life is strikingly clear for young people and their families who live it every day. The level of control (i.e. the HbA$_{1c}$ young people achieve) speaks volumes about where they position themselves in terms of how intensive a regimen they are prepared to adhere to routinely. The goals of health professionals are focused primarily on maintaining or improving diabetes control to prevent long-term complications, while paying lip service to quality of life. Parents, despite valuing quality of life, will also most often view the prevention of long-term complications as their highest priority. However, there is a dramatic variation in the priorities that children and young people assign to diabetes control and quality of life.

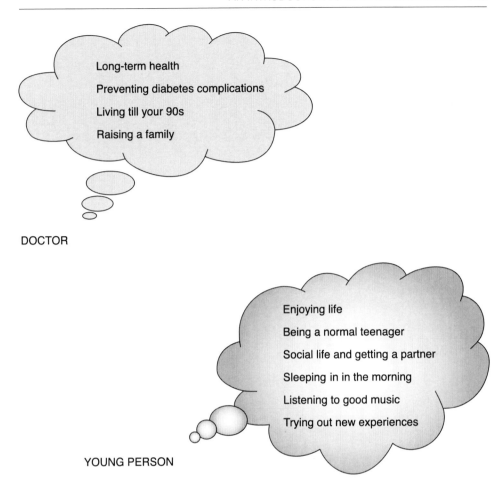

FIGURE 8.3 Priorities

Patterns of control

Health professionals have tended to have monolithic concepts of 'poor control' in diabetes, particularly in teenagers. The standard conceptualisation of the poorly controlled adolescent with diabetes is one of a young person who is non-adherent to insulin, blood glucose monitoring and dietary regimens, resulting in high HbA$_{1c}$ and possibly recurrent episodes of diabetic ketoacidosis (DKA) (Henderson, 1991). The adolescent is generally seen to be unmotivated, potentially poorly educated about their diabetes and chaotic in their dietary, insulin and blood glucose habits. Postulated causes of this are assumed to be a combination of family and social problems, adolescent 'rebellion' and psychological problems related to having diabetes (Liss *et al.*, 1998). There are variable degrees of evidence to support this view, as discussed elsewhere in this book (*see*, for example, Chapter 6).

However, the majority of patients with high HbA$_{1c}$ do not have recurrent DKA. The prevalence of recurrent DKA in adolescents is low (Edge *et al.*, 1999). In fact, approximately 20–40 young people internationally maintain high HbA$_{1c}$ values, e.g. > 8.5% (de Beaufort *et al.*, 2007; Gerstl *et al.*, 2008), well above that regarded as optimal for prevention of diabetic complications. Yet our understandings of 'poor control' in adolescence tend to conflate high HbA$_{1c}$ and recurrent DKA.

Further, while we recognise hypoglycaemia as a major issue in diabetes control, it features rarely within our conceptualisations of poor control in adolescence. Excessive hypoglycaemia associated with a very low HbA$_{1c}$ (e.g. < 5.0%) is a dangerous version of diabetes control that is clinically seen not infrequently but is rarely conceptualised as 'poor diabetes control'. Conversely, while the majority of teenagers with a high HbA$_{1c}$ or recurrent DKA do not have major problems with hypoglycaemia episodes, some young people experience highly variable blood glucose, running from hyper- to hypoglycaemia most days. Such young people may have relatively 'good' HbA$_{1c}$ values. We now recognise that the latter pattern of high glucose variability is almost certainly associated with poorer cardiovascular outcomes independently of HbA$_{1c}$.

Thus, we have three key issues to factor into our concepts of control:
1. the overall level of glycaemic control, as measured by HbA$_{1c}$
2. hypoglycaemic episodes
3. admissions to hospital for DKA.

The balance point a young person feels comfortable with determines the pattern of diabetes control they manifest – and that we see as health professionals – in their measured HbA$_{1c}$, in the number of hypoglycaemic episodes and in admissions for DKA. To illustrate this, let us return to the 35 adherence points we identified as potentially needed to control diabetes carefully and at a satisfactory level. One needs to ask a number of questions:
- What proportion of young people achieves such a large number of adherence points each day?
- What do most young people achieve?
- How many are actually necessary?

We don't have clear answers to these questions. Some hypotheses are presented here.

Max's story (*see* Case Study 1) presents a typical history for many young people we see in adolescent diabetes clinics.

Case study 1: Max, aged 14 years

Max was seen in the adolescent diabetes clinic. He had had diabetes for 7 years and his HbA$_{1c}$ had been running at approximately 10%–12% for the past 2 years, worsening dramatically from previous good control from the time that Max took over most of his diabetes care, at around 12 years old. His insulin regimen was two daily injections of Humalog Mix25, with a total prescribed dose of 1.6 U/kg/day. His body mass index was on the 50th centile. He reported rare blood glucose monitoring, only with suspected hypoglycaemic episodes, although he had not recognised a 'hypo' or measured capillary blood glucose in the previous 3 months. He denied symptoms of significant hyperglycaemia, although he had not been undertaking urine ketone testing. He had not been admitted to hospital for diabetes since diagnosis at the age of 7. The diabetes team had become increasingly concerned about Max and had attempted to implement a number of changes over the previous 24 months, including intensive education sessions, complication screening (he had no evidence of microvascular complications) and intensification of clinic visits, with no effect. The diabetes educators reported that Max's diabetes knowledge was in fact quite good. Max had resisted attempts to intensify his insulin regimen, being particularly reluctant to take a lunchtime injection at school, and had rejected suggestions of referral to the clinic psychologist.

Max's HbA$_{1c}$, at 10%–12%, clearly signifies very poor diabetes control, placing him at high risk for microvascular complications in the intermediate and long term. Yet looking at the other elements of control, he has no hypoglycaemic episodes and he has not been admitted for DKA for years. He has one element of poor control, but not the others. If we calculate how many daily adherence points he achieves, we find the answer to be only two to three per day. No blood glucose testing, little or no focus on diet, no hypoglycaemic episodes with exercise, therefore no need to worry about diabetes with exercise. To the doctor and nurse in clinic, Max clearly has very poor diabetes control due to very poor or minimal adherence with his prescribed diabetes regimen.

Imagine we now turn to Max and ask him about his quality of life. He tells us that doing no blood glucose testing, ignoring the diabetes diet, never having hypoglycaemic episodes and taking only two injections per day means that diabetes hardly interferes with his daily life at all. His friends don't know about his diabetes, as his injections are all done at home. The realisation dawns on us that, to all appearances, Max only 'has diabetes' at the time of his morning injection and his dinner injection.

If we tried to see things through Max's eyes, or asked him how well he controlled diabetes in his life, we may come to think that Max has superb control of his diabetes in that he's entirely in charge of diabetes: it interferes minimally with his life and it doesn't set him apart from other young people. Indeed, Max probably has a quality of life no different to any other teenager. The only thing that interferes with this is the increasing level of worry expressed by his parents and the healthcare team.

It is important to recognise here that Max has had diabetes for some years, is knowledgeable about his diabetes and does not have chaotic or uncontrolled glucose levels (high or low) or admissions to hospitals. Indeed, he probably has relatively stable blood glucose levels. How do we explain this pattern? How does this fit with the clear evidence from Max's HbA$_{1c}$ that he has poor diabetes control that will lead inevitably to long-term complications? Pondering this question we should come to the question that we need to ask: when we think about *control*, whose control do we mean and exactly what is being controlled? We need to recognise that *control* for patients may mean things other than metabolic control.

In clinic, we would need to recognise that Max's behaviour and pattern of diabetes control is actually extremely common and in fact it is a skilful set of behaviours adopted by young people with a long history of diabetes and a relatively good knowledge base. We believe that it is the commonest form of poor glycaemic control in teenagers, much more common than recurrent DKA.

How is Max achieving his version of diabetes control? The answer is by being carefully adherent to a diabetes regimen *of his own choosing*, by carefully using the body's ability to sense blood glucose within very wide limits to maintain blood glucose levels between 10 and 25 mmol, and by having a fairly regular daily routine without significant exercise. The diabetes regimen is usually the minimum number of injections that the clinic will tolerate, and careful poor control is possible with two, three or four injections per day, although most commonly with two. The only way to avoid blood glucose testing and avoid hypoglycaemia is to carefully run blood glucose moderately high, e.g. between 10 and 20 mmol mostly, with occasionally higher or lower excursions. This will reset hypo awareness thresholds, so that young people feel hypo at any blood glucose less than around 8 mmol/L, thus almost always avoiding hypoglycaemia. Sensitivity to bodily perceptions will allow young people to identify blood glucose over 20 mmol/L.

Concepts of purposeful, 'careful' but poor control sit poorly within our standard medical understandings of chronic disease control, which tend to assume that poor control results from deficits – lack of education, lack of interest, lack of ability to adhere or possibility more complex problems, including family problems or mental health issues.

However, this careful pattern of poor control requires skill, planning, good internal body perceptions and quite careful adherence. It is the exact opposite of the standard assumption about 'chaotic' or 'non-adherent' adolescent poor control. For this reason, many of our traditional approaches to poor control – such as 'a good talking to', improved education, more intensive clinic supervision, or referral against the young person's wishes to a psychologist or social worker – are entirely inappropriate and are highly unlikely to succeed or to be acceptable to patients, as they start from incorrect assumptions.

The appropriate responses to careful poor control must arise from an understanding of why young people adopt this pattern. Health professionals tend to assume a rationality in patients that matches our own; that is, assuming that failure to prioritise achieving the best glycaemic control reflects a 'problem' rather than an active choice. As noted, we assume these problems relate to poor education, teenage apathy, chaotic lifestyle or problems in the family. The latter is a particular trap for child health professionals, whose focus on the wider social context of children's lives often leads them to be quick to identify family problems as the cause of young people's problems. Yet in our experience young people who adopt careful poor control behaviours have few of these problems. For them, their behaviours simply reflect the low priority they assign to diabetes control compared with a very high priority placed on preserving quality of life. Such young people place the control versus quality of life balance point firmly on the side of normal life.

This should make us revise our terminology when we speak about control. Glycaemic control is certainly related to HbA_{1c} and hypoglycaemia and recurrent DKA. However, we should reserve the term *diabetes control* for a wider concept, one that includes the patients' perspective and aspects of quality of life in addition to medical aspects of control.

If young people with careful poor control represent one end of the spectrum, prioritising quality of life almost entirely over glycaemic control, what about the other end of the spectrum? It could be argued that those who almost entirely prioritise diabetes control over quality of life have a different pattern of poor diabetes control. They may or may not have good glycaemic control, poor glycaemic control in this instance being an abnormally low HbA_{1c} with an excessive amount of hypos. However, they are also highly likely to have poor quality of life and psychological distress, such as depression (*see* Chapter 3).

There is probably a range of other clear patterns of poor control of diabetes in young people. Recurrent DKA and high HbA_{1c} due to insulin withholding are just two. These will not be discussed in detail here: suffice it to say that they are both patterns of diabetic control where glycaemic control is subservient to young people's other priorities – either maintaining a slim figure (insulin withholding) or other psychological issues (recurrent DKA).

FROM PATTERN RECOGNITION TO ACTION

The recognition that a young person's pattern of poor diabetes control is very largely a personal response to dilemmas over the priority balance between glycaemic control and quality of life allows us to formulate a response that is highly likely to be effective. If there is a mismatch between action and control pattern, the intervention is unlikely to help the young person improve their glycaemic control. There are undoubtedly young people in whom poor diabetes control reflects significant psychopathology, and who fit poorly into the schema outlined here. They are most commonly those with recurrent DKA or those with excessive hypos and very rarely those with careful poor control.

Recognising the young person's specific pattern of poor control is the first step. The second is to understand why they do what they do; that is, to understand what their main priorities are, what their health beliefs are, and to which elements of their regimen they are routinely adherent. The third step is checking with them what level of HbA$_{1c}$ they would like to run. My experience is that most young people with careful poor control actually desire good HbA$_{1c}$ levels and rate glycaemic control as important, but don't prioritise achieving this. They do see poor control as a problem for them, and they have an intellectual belief that glycaemic control is desirable. However, achieving a good HbA$_{1c}$ is a low priority for them. In quite a typical adolescent fashion, contemporary goals are prioritised over future problems.

This information can help the health professional work with the young person to allow them to achieve their high-priority goals (i.e. high quality of life), while helping them achieve their low-priority goal (which is our high-priority goal) of improving glycaemic control. However, this almost certainly requires some negotiated intensification of regimen on the part of the young person. Motivational enhancement techniques offer very useful ways to begin this process – to help them examine their priorities, work out whether poor control is a problem for them and work with them to help change occur and to maintain these changes. Chapters 11 and 12 describe these approaches in detail in relation to engaging young people in the process of change.

SUMMARY

Modern intensive diabetes regimens may significantly impact on quality of life and force young people to choose a personal balance point between regimen work/adherence and enjoyment of life. Diabetes control should be understood as comprising quality of life in addition to achieving glycaemic control. Health professionals frequently regard 'poor diabetes control' in crude and monolithic ways, and see young people with poor control as non-adherent, chaotic, poorly informed or distressed. Frequently, they are none of these. Instead, many young people skilfully adhere to a regimen of their own choosing, one that prioritises quality of life over glycaemic control – a careful poor control pattern. Other patterns of poor control reflect different balances and the outcomes of a different prioritisation process. Approaches to improving poor diabetes control require an understanding of the highly personal nature of patterns of poor control, an understanding of health beliefs and priorities and the use of motivational and solution-focused techniques to help young people achieve and maintain change towards improved glycaemic control.

REFERENCES

Betts PR, Jefferson IG, Swift PG. Diabetes care in childhood and adolescence. *Diabet Med.* 2002; **19**(Suppl. 4): 61–5.

De Beaufort CE, Swift PG, Skinner CT, *et al.* Continuing stability of center differences in pediatric diabetes care: do advances in diabetes treatment improve outcome? The Hvidoere Study Group on Childhood Diabetes. *Diabetes Care.* 2007; **30**(9): 2245–50.

Edge JA, Ford-Adams ME, Dunger DB. Causes of death in children with insulin dependent diabetes 1990–96. *Arch Dis Child.* 1999; **81**(4): 318–23.

Gerstl EM, Rabl W, Rosenbauer J, *et al.* Metabolic control as reflected by HbA1c in children, adolescents and young adults with type-1 diabetes mellitus: combined longitudinal analysis including 27,035 patients from 207 centers in Germany and Austria during the last decade. *Eur J Pediatr.* 2008; **167**(4): 447–53.

Gosden C, Edge JA, Holt RI, *et al.* The fifth UK paediatric diabetes services survey: meeting guidelines and recommendations? *Arch Dis Child.* 2010; **95**(10): 837–40.

Henderson G. The psychosocial treatment of recurrent diabetic ketoacidosis: an interdisciplinary team approach. *Diabetes Educ.* 1991; **17**(2): 119–23.

Liss DS, Waller DA, Kennard BD, *et al.* Psychiatric illness and family support in children and adolescents with diabetic ketoacidosis: a controlled study. *J Am Acad Child Adolesc Psychiatry.* 1998; **37**(5): 536–44.

White NH, Cleary PA, Dahms W, *et al.* Beneficial effects of intensive therapy of diabetes during adolescence: outcomes after the conclusion of the Diabetes Control and Complications Trial (DCCT). *J Pediatr.* 2001; **139**(6): 804–12.

CHAPTER 9

Structured education for diabetes

Rebecca Thompson

INTRODUCTION

As identified in Chapter 1, the number of young people with diabetes is increasing. At the time of writing, there is no 'cure' for diabetes; therefore, finding ways to help children and young people cope with its demands and to improve outcomes is essential. Education is considered to be key to this and has been described as the ongoing process of facilitating knowledge and skills needed to perform diabetes self-care, manage crises and to make lifestyle changes to successfully manage the disease (Funnel *et al.*, 2010; Swift, 2009). Although national paediatric guidelines emphasise the importance of education, structured education of children and young people with diabetes lags behind that developed for adults, with no agreed standardised structured education package available in the United Kingdom.

The following chapter will explore the rationale of education provision and review available standards. It will then consider the kind of specification education packages children and young people should have and, finally, how the effectiveness of such resources may be evaluated.

THE IMPORTANCE OF AN EDUCATIONAL PROGRAMME

The importance of educating people with diabetes was recognised within 2 years of the introduction of insulin. Joslin *et al.* (1922) stated that every insulin-treated patient had to be properly educated to be able to manage their own care. However, despite such early recommendations, it has taken 50 years for the beneficial effects of patient education to be finally proven, repositioning it from being an ad hoc event to one that is central to successful self-management (Assal *et al.*, 1985; Lucas and Walker, 2004).

Recently, there has been much attention paid to education, with national and international guidelines all emphasising the need for structured patient education. In the United Kingdom, documents from the Department of Health (DoH, 2001, 2004, 2007) support self-care and empowerment as crucial aspects of any high-quality diabetes service, with the central pillars being patient-centred care and timely access to specialist education and support. Similarly, the National Institute for Clinical Excellence technology appraisal (NICE, 2003) on patient education models recommended that structured patient education should be made available at the time of initial diagnosis and then as required on an ongoing basis, according to formal, regular assessment of need.

For adults living with diabetes, there are a number of recognised education programmes, including:

- Dose Adjustment for Normal Eating (DAFNE, 2002)
- DESMOND (Diabetes Education and Self Management for Ongoing and Newly Diagnosed) (Davies *et al.*, 2008)
- Diabetes X-PERT (structured education for people with diabetes) (www. xperthealth.org.uk/).

For children and adolescents living with type 1 diabetes, many diabetes centres in the United Kingdom offer education. However, there is no nationally agreed standardised education package. In addition, little attention has been given to the education needs of children and adolescents with type 2 diabetes.

Considering the evidence

There have been a number of literature reviews examining the effectiveness of educational interventions specifically for children and young people living with diabetes. The effect of education on diabetes knowledge is unclear, with some studies reporting a small to medium beneficial effect on diabetes outcomes (Couch *et al.*, 2008; Hampson *et al.*, 2001). A distinction has been made between the traditional education approach and those that address psychosocial issues arising from living with diabetes. The evidence suggests that educational interventions may improve diabetes knowledge but are not consistently helpful in improving metabolic control (Grey, 2000). In contrast, psychosocial interventions that include coping-skills training and peer support and that demonstrate the interrelatedness of the various aspects of diabetes management have been shown to improve adjustment and sometimes metabolic control (Grey, 2000; Hampson *et al.*, 2001).

Randomised studies have been unable to demonstrate that education programmes are an effective intervention for those young people with very poorly controlled diabetes (Gage *et al.*, 2004; Murphy *et al.*, 2006). These results offer support to the view that poor metabolic control is not merely a reflection of poor knowledge. However, the evidence suggests that *combining* education with psychological approaches can achieve engagement, motivation and long-term change for these young people who have not responded to other approaches (Hampson *et al.*, 2001).

AVAILABLE NATIONAL AND INTERNATIONAL STANDARDS
The international standards for diabetes education

The revised standards developed by the International Diabetes Federation (IDF, 2003) consultative section on diabetes education (*see* Box 9.1) provide a basis to establish, evaluate and improve diabetes education. It is envisaged that these standards can be used to benchmark the quality of care delivered both by organisations and individual educators. The standards are organised into structure, process and outcome, with each of these having detailed indicators.

BOX 9.1 International standards for diabetes education, 2003

- There is documented evidence of organisational/institutional support for education as an integral part of diabetes care.
- One person will be identified to be responsible for the organisation and administration of the diabetes service in such a way that the process and outcome standards can be met.
- Physical space and education resources are conducive to learning and based on individual/community needs.
- An advisory committee is established to ensure that the views and values of all stakeholders are represented in the ongoing planning and delivery of diabetes education.
- Teamwork and communication are evident among those providing diabetes education and management.
- Personnel involved in diabetes education have a sound clinical understanding of diabetes and are knowledgeable about teaching and learning skills and diabetes self-management practices.
- The competence and performance of personnel involved in diabetes education is reviewed at least annually.
- Professional staff in the diabetes service are appointed on a permanent basis, not on a rotational basis.
- Diabetes education covers topics based on individual assessment and fosters acquisition of knowledge leading to self-management of diabetes.
- Relationships are fostered with available community resources, such as diabetes associations, blind society and social services.

- Diabetes education is based on the ongoing learner-centred needs assessments of individuals and/or communities.
- Plans for individual diabetes education and diabetes education programmes are learner centred and subject to ongoing review and modification.
- Implementation of diabetes education is learner centred and facilitates cognitive learning, behaviour change and self-management and is extended to families, caregivers and communities where appropriate.
- Education is provided in a professional and ethical manner and is learner centred and evidence based where possible.
- The diabetes education service will be recognised by and will be accessible to the community.
- The effectiveness and quality of the education will be annually assessed, linked to outcomes and the services will be reviewed on the basis of the assessment.
- Educational and clinical research are undertaken to provide an evidence base for practice.
- Communities are aware of the risk factors for the development of diabetes and actions that may delay the onset of diabetes mellitus and its potential complications.
- Communities are aware of the different types of diabetes mellitus and the needs and support available for individuals living with diabetes.
- People with diabetes will understand, depending on their individual capabilities, how diabetes affects their bodies and the significance of maintaining a healthy lifestyle.
- Individuals with diabetes make informed decisions and take deliberate actions towards healthy living with diabetes.
- The physical, psychological and emotional health of the individual will be improved.

With specific regard to paediatric education, the standards reproduced in Box 9.1 describe how the initial and ongoing needs assessments should recognise the diversity and changing needs of children, that personnel providing education to this age range need to have training and expertise specific to the special and changing needs of childhood and adolescence, and how diabetes-related absence from school should be minimised.

Structured Patient Education in Diabetes

The Structured Patient Education in Diabetes patient education working group agreed on a set of quality standards for education programmes (DoH and DUK, 2005). The report recognises a gap in the provision of education for children and young people and identifies key aspects of a high-quality, structured education programme that fulfils NICE guidelines (NICE, 2004). The philosophy that underpins the programme is that it is evidence based, dynamic and flexible to the needs of the individual and users should be involved in its ongoing development. In addition, education programmes should have specific aims, and learning objectives should be shared with patients' carers and families.

Four key criteria are identified as being essential within an effective education programme:

1. a structured, written curriculum
2. trained educators
3. quality assurance
4. audit.

It is recommended that local teams work towards these criteria and aim to ensure that any education programme meets these standards.

Canadian Diabetes Association: clinical practice guidelines for the prevention and management of diabetes

The principles underlying these guidelines (CDA, 2008) are:

- the tailoring of essential components of self-management education to individual needs and circumstances
- the provision of education in a group setting, alongside others who share the same condition
- feedback following intervention
- a psychological emphasis on interventions
- inclusion of those providing medical interventions.

While there is no specific paediatric guidance, the guidelines describe how programmes must be individualised according to the type of diabetes, current state of metabolic stability, learning ability, capacity for change, motivation and resources. When indicated, interventions that target the families' abilities to cope with stress or diabetes-related conflict should be considered, with recognition that education within the home setting can be effective for adolescents with type 1 diabetes.

International Society of Pediatric and Adolescent Diabetes clinical practice consensus guidelines: diabetes education

The International Society of Pediatric and Adolescent Diabetes (ISPAD) consensus guidelines (Swift *et al.*, 2009) describe how every child and young person has a right to comprehensive, expert, structured education, which should empower them and their families to take control of their diabetes.

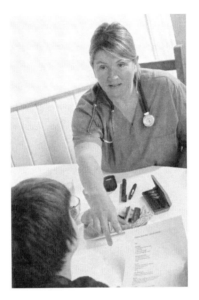

The diabetes educator gives advice on nutrition

In order to put the four key criteria outlined into practice, the ISPAD recommend:
- Structured education should be available to all people with diabetes at the time of initial diagnosis, or when it is appropriate for them, and then as required on an ongoing basis, based on a formal, regular individual assessment of need.
- Education should be provided by an appropriately trained interdisciplinary team – the team should have a sound understanding of the principles governing teaching and learning.
- Interdisciplinary teams providing education should include, as a minimum, a diabetes specialist nurse and a dietitian.
- Sessions should be held in a location accessible to individuals and families, whether in the community or at the inpatient centre.
- Educational programmes should use a variety of teaching techniques, adapted wherever possible to meet the different needs, personal choices and learning styles of young people with diabetes and parents, as well as local models of care.

National standards for diabetes self-management education

A task force jointly convened by the American Association of Diabetes Educators and the American Diabetes Association agreed on a consensus of 10 national standards (*see* Box 9.2) designed to define quality programmes and to assist educators in providing evidence-based programmes. The overall objectives of diabetes self-management education are described as supporting informed decision-making, self-care behaviours, problem-solving and active collaboration with the healthcare team and to improve clinical outcomes, health status and quality of life (Funnell *et al.*, 2010).

BOX 9.2 National standards for diabetes self-management education

Structure

1. The diabetes self-management education (DSME) entity will have documentation of its organisational structure, mission statement and goals and will recognise and support quality DSME as an integral component of diabetes care.
2. The DSME entity shall appoint an advisory group to promote quality, including representatives from the health professions, people with diabetes, the community and other stakeholders.
3. The DSME entity will determine the diabetes educational needs of the target population(s) and identify resources necessary to meet these needs.
4. A coordinator will be designated to oversee the planning, implementation and evaluation of diabetes self-management education. The coordinator will have academic or experiential preparation in chronic disease care and education and in programme management.

Process

5. DSME will be provided by one or more instructors. The instructors will have recent educational and experiential preparation in education and diabetes management or be a certified diabetes educator.
6. A written curriculum reflecting current evidence and guidelines, with criteria for evaluating outcomes, will serve as the framework for the DSME entity. Assessed needs of the individual with pre-diabetes and diabetes will determine the content to be provided.
7. The participant and the instructor will collaboratively develop an individual assessment and education plan to direct the selection of appropriate educational interventions and self-management support strategies. This assessment and education plan and the intervention and outcomes will be documented in the education record.
8. The participant and instructor(s) will collaboratively develop a personalised

follow-up plan for ongoing self-management support. The patient's outcomes and goals and the plan for ongoing self-management support will be communicated to the referring provider.

Outcomes

9. The DSME entity will measure attainment of patient-defined goals and patient outcomes at regular intervals using appropriate measurement techniques to evaluate the effectiveness of the educational intervention.

10. The DSME entity will measure the effectiveness of the education process and determine opportunities for improvement using a written continuous quality improvement plan that describes and documents a systematic review of the entities process and outcome data.

WHAT SHOULD AN EDUCATIONAL PROGRAMME LOOK LIKE?

Learning-needs assessment

Most of the standards recommend that the design of an education package is based upon formal, regular assessment of need. These learning-needs assessments can be used both to clarify the direction to be taken for educational planning and in auditing how successful the education has been.

The patient education working group (DoH and DUK, 2005) developed four themes around which patients educational needs might be assessed. These included (i) contextual data such as age, gender and relationship with other family members and carers; (ii) previous diabetes education; (iii) personal models of illness; and (iv) self-empowered behaviour.

In relation to paediatrics, healthcare professionals need to have a clear understanding of the special and changing needs of young people and their families as they grow through the different stages of life. The needs of children and adolescents will obviously alter over the years and, clearly, age and developmental status are powerful contextual variables that influence both the child's understanding of how their own body works and their involvement in diabetes self-management.

Educational programmes need to accommodate the needs of children and parents at various ages and developmental stages. For example, preschool children are totally dependent on their parents and care providers; therefore, education needs to be adapted to the needs of these adults. The focus will change for an 8-year-old, who may be expected to test their blood glucose or give an occasional injection with supervision. There may be a complete shift in emphasis for the adolescent, who may be expected to learn to take responsibility for some tasks and take on some shared responsibility for decision-making with their parents or carers. There is no consensus within the literature or within clinical practice as to when or at what age children with type 1 diabetes should assume self-management responsibilities.

It is clear that diabetes education needs to be adaptable and personalised so that it is appropriate to each individual's age, stage of diabetes, maturity and lifestyle, as well as being culturally sensitive and delivered at a pace to suit individual needs.

Curriculum

Whilst national and international standards (as previously discussed) describe the structure, process and outcomes of diabetes education, there is less specification on the curriculum or the content of diabetes education programmes. What is clear is that learning needs are going to vary depending on the timing of the educational delivery and on the type of diabetes diagnosed.

ISPAD-published guidelines (Swift *et al.*, 2009) can be used as a template with which to develop an appropriate educational curriculum for children and young people with diabetes. Topics are divided into two levels. The initial level covers the survival skills needed at diagnosis, including an explanation as to how the diagnosis has been made, the need for immediate insulin, basic dietetic advice, what glucose is (and does) and practical skills such as injections and blood glucose monitoring. The second level of the educational curriculum includes such topics as pathophysiology and classification; insulin secretion, insulin action and profiles, nutrition, exercise, problem-solving and goal-setting.

There is little published information specifically related to the curriculum for children and adolescents with type 2 diabetes (Atkinson and Radjenovic, 2007). While many of the national standards for diabetes self-management education may be applicable, the curriculum is likely to have common themes but a different emphasis. Education will need to have potential emphasis on willingness to lose or maintain weight, to exercise and to be willing to change eating behaviours. These lifestyle issues should be included in programmes designed to raise awareness and improve understanding of the disease process of type 2 diabetes, blood glucose levels, medication and their side effects.

Trained educators

Joint documents from the Department of Health and Diabetes UK (DoH and DUK, 2005) highlight the importance of structured training of educators and trainers involved in delivering patient-education programmes. However, members of paediatric and adolescent diabetes teams in the United Kingdom have a varying amount of input in relation to age-specific and developmental milestones for children and adolescents, and there is no current consensus across the United Kingdom to allow uniformity for roles and qualifications for different members of those teams to deliver structured patient education.

There is increasing international interest in exploring the possibility of the diabetes educator role. Countries such as the United States, Canada and Australia already use diabetes educators, where the role is well established and defined. These individuals are healthcare professionals from a variety of disciplines, whose roles are to focus on helping people with diabetes achieve behaviour-change goals which lead to better clinical outcomes and improved health status (American Association of Diabetes Educators). Diabetes educators apply knowledge and skills in the biological and social sciences, communication, counselling and education to provide self-management training. Some countries have developed rigorous accreditation procedures involving specific education programmes, mentorship and certification procedures, such as the Certified Diabetes Educator (CDE) credential in the United States. Chapter 10 discusses these roles in greater detail.

Challenges to structured education delivery

One of the constant challenges in delivering education or training is finding the right balance between diabetes and other priorities in the lives of children and young people. A good example of this is deciding when education packages should be delivered. Education groups that run during the working day of the healthcare professional often conflict with education, causing the young person to miss school. Alternatively, evening and weekends may conflict with social activities that a young person engages in (and most likely will prioritise over their attendance at a diabetes education session).

Practical challenges include locating suitable space for holding structured education groups. Many hospitals have limited facilities dedicated to teaching. Education groups are rarely held at the same time as the standard clinic appointments. While it is recognised that there are challenges to running group education alongside the diabetes clinic, running them at different times results in young people having to find more 'diabetes time' in their lives and parents taking additional time off work.

In the United Kingdom, much of the structured education is being delivered by diabetes specialist nurses, with differing levels of support from other members of the diabetes team. Nurses working in isolation in small diabetes teams may struggle to deliver structured education, while managing ever-expanding caseloads of patients. However, national standards (Funnell *et al.*, 2010; IDF, 2003) recognise the need for multidisciplinary teams to achieve optimal educational intervention, though cost issues can compromise this provision. In some countries, the cost of providing education is covered by healthcare insurance. In the United Kingdom, proposed changes to national tariffs and 'payment by results' recognise that structured education is an important component of care and changes in payment systems may enable a more multidisciplinary approach to diabetes education in the future.

Agreeing to participate in structured education requires the young person to see diabetes as a priority in their lives. If a young person does not want to change the way they manage their diabetes, they are unlikely to agree to attend. Here, healthcare professionals need to develop the skills that they can use to engage these young people. For example, psychological approaches such as motivational interviewing may be integrated into routine follow-up sessions. Education delivery needs to be interactive rather than didactic and to use real situations relevant to the young person. To be most effective, sessions need to include not only the child or young person but also people involved in caring for them, be a continuous process and be repeated as required (Funnell *et al.*, 2010).

EVALUATING THE EFFECTIVENESS OF PATIENT EDUCATION
What and how?

The aim of patient education is for people with diabetes (or their carers) to improve their knowledge, skills and confidence, enabling them to become experts at managing their (or their child's) diabetes on a day-to-day basis. Given this aim, what criteria should be used to judge the effectiveness of a structured education package?

Managing diabetes within a full and active life is challenging, both for children and for young people. Therefore, measuring medical outcomes such as HbA_{1c} is important in diabetes. Despite parental support and 'expert' education, many children and young people struggle to control their diabetes, with only 16.2% of children in the United Kingdom achieving an HbA_{1c} of less than 7.5% (< 59 mmol/mol). It has been reported that nearly 30% of those with records submitted have a high-risk HbA_{1c} of greater than 9.5% (NHS, 2010). Recently evaluated structured education programmes have been unable to demonstrate a significant improvement in HbA_{1c} (Chaney *et al.*, 2010; Murphy *et al.*, 2007; Waller *et al.*, 2008)

Many of the local structured education packages in the United Kingdom use quiz-based assessment at the end of the session to assess patient knowledge, but there is no standard template to assist assessment of patient knowledge and skills. If we want to improve HbA_{1c} and believe education is the key, how do we assess objectively what children and their families know to then enable us, as healthcare professionals, to provide the right education to develop young people's knowledge and skills and for this to then be put into practice?

The team at the Children's Hospital in Los Angeles have developed an eight-stage competency system to be able to assess skills and knowledge within diabetes management. The eight stages are outlined in Table 9.1.

TABLE 9.1 Competency Level Scale, from 1 to 8 (Kaufman *et al.*, 2001)

Competency	Characteristics	Level
Safety	Initial information, injections, blood testing, treatment for hypoglycaemia	1
Basics	Blood glucose targets, actions for levels out of target, glucagon, action of different types of insulin, diet and carbohydrate	2
Carbohydrate management	Determine quantity of carbohydrates in food, use of plan for carbohydrate intake	3
Correction	How to correct blood glucose out of target	4
Daily changes	Decision-making about changes in daily routine, adjusting insulin and carbohydrate intake	5
Base dose adjustment	Making base dose adjustments, review blood glucose values to observe overall effects of treatments	6
Advanced diabetes management	Understand hormone pathways and food absorption; know about strategies to reduce complications	7
Maximised control, basal and bolus therapy	Independence in multiple daily injections/continuous subcutaneous insulin infusion to maximise control, flexibility and freedom	8

In a study reported by Kaufman *et al.* (2001), the competencies outlined in Table 9.1 were used by the healthcare team to assess readiness for pump therapy, with families needing to demonstrate skills and knowledge at a minimum of competency level 5. Through the use of this measure, in conjunction with starting insulin pump therapy, a significant and sustained reduction in HbA1c over a 2-year period was achieved.

There needs to be further exploration as to whether a competency-based tool can be used to measure the effectiveness of structured education within paediatric diabetes. Healthcare professionals need to collaborate with specialists within education to formulate appropriate and reliable methods of evaluation (Assal *et al.*, 1985) that can be used in addition to measuring changes in HbA_{1c}.

Accreditation

There is currently no formal accreditation body in the United Kingdom to accredit national or local patient education programmes, and each of the current programmes is individual in respect to its curriculum and how it is delivered. While most pilot programmes appear to increase patient satisfaction (compared with no education), positive biomedical outcomes in the short term are inconclusive. There is a recognised need for further research in relation to educating children and their families about diabetes, where the design is based upon an explicit hypothesis and educational theory and the range of outcomes is evaluated after long follow-up intervals.

Quality assurance

There is no standard template that can be used by local paediatric and adolescent diabetes teams to assist assessment of patient knowledge and skills, yet the structure of quality assurance is crucial to ensure that this is a rigorous process. Programmes like DAFNE and DESMOND have contributed to the development of robust quality assurance processes and are enabling learning to be shared about how they can be used effectively. Quality assurance should have clear, written standards that can be monitored, regularly reviewed and updated.

BOX 9.3 The quality assurance process should be made up of three main elements

1. Development of a defined programme. This should have a clear content, structure, curriculum and underlying philosophy. The training programme for educators should itself be included within the quality assurance process
2. Defined quality assurance tools that are based on the structure of the programme, and identify a set of observable behaviours required to deliver the programme
3. An internal and external process to assess the delivery and organisation of the programme.

The Quality Institute for Self Management Education and Training[1] is an independent verifying body set up in 2009. It has begun to develop diabetes structured patient education certification and standards. While the aim is to assure the delivery of consistently high-quality diabetes self-management education within local systems of care, the draft standards at the time of writing are currently out for consultation.

SUMMARY

There is still insufficient evidence to recommend the use of one particular educational programme. It is accepted that well-designed educational intervention trials are needed in the United Kingdom, with large sample sizes and multicentre collaboration. While there are many structured education packages that are currently in development in the United Kingdom, a small number are being undertaken as multicentre randomised control trials. These include:

- CHOICE (CarboHydrate, Insulin Collaborative Education) (Chaney *et al.*, 2010).

---

1 With funding support from the Department of Health.

- Kick-Off (Kids in Control of Food) (Waller *et al.*, 2008).
- FACTS (Families, Adolescents and Children's Teamwork Study) (Murphy *et al.*, 2007)
- CASCADE (Child and Adolescent Structured Competencies Approach to Diabetes Education, Christie *et al.*, 2009).

REFERENCES

Assal JP, Mühlhauser I, Pernet A, *et al.* Patient education as the basis for diabetes care in clinical practice and research. *Diabetologia.* 1985; **28**(8): 602–13.

Atkinson A, Radjenovic D. Meeting quality standards for self-management education in pediatric type 2 diabetes. *Diabetes Spectrum.* 2007; **20**(1): 40–6.

Canadian Diabetes Association (CDA). Clinical Practice Guidelines for the prevention and management of diabetes in Canada. *Can J Diabetes.* 2008; **32**(Suppl. 1); 1–215.

Chaney D, Coates V, Shevlin M. Running a complex educational intervention for adolescents with type 1 diabetes: lessons learnt. *J Diabetes Nurs.* 2010; **14**(10): 370–9.

Christie, D, Strange, V, Allen, E. *et al.* Maximising engagement, motivation, and long term change in a structured intensive education programme in diabetes for children and their families; Child and Adolescent Structured Competencies Approach to Diabetes Education (CASCADE), BMC PEDIATRICS, 2009; **9**: 57.

Couch R, Jetha M, Dryden DM, *et al.* Diabetes education for children with type 1 diabetes mellitus and their families. *Evid Rep Technol Assess (Full Rep).* 2008; (166): 1–144.

DAFNE Study Group. Training in flexible, intensive insulin management to enable dietary freedom in people with type 1 diabetes: dose adjustment for normal eating (DAFNE) randomised controlled trial. *BMJ.* 2002; **325**(7367): 746.

Davies MJ, Heller S, Skinner TC, *et al.* Effectiveness of the diabetes education and self management for ongoing and newly diagnosed (DESMOND) programme for people with newly diagnosed type 2 diabetes: cluster randomised controlled trial. *BMJ.* 2008; **336**(7642): 491–5.

Department of Health (DoH). *Diabetes Service Framework for Diabetes: standards.* London: DoH publications; 2001.

Department of Health (DoH). *Children's National Service Framework for Children, Young People and Maternity Services: core standards.* London: DoH publications; 2004.

Department of Health (DoH). *Making Every Young Person with Diabetes Matter.* London: DoH publications; 2007.

Department of Health and Diabetes UK (DoH and DUK). *Structured Patient Education in Diabetes: report for the patient education working group.* London: DoH Publications; 2005.

Funnell MM, Brown TL, Childs BP, *et al.* National standards for diabetes self-management education. *Diabetes Care.* 2010; **33**(Suppl. 1): S89–96.

Gage H, Hampson S, Skinner TC, *et al.* Educational and psychosocial programmes for adolescents with diabetes: approaches, outcomes and cost-effectiveness. *Patient Educ Couns.* 2004; **53**(3): 333–46.

Grey M. Interventions for children with diabetes and their families. *Ann Rev Nurs Res.* 2000; **18**: 149–70.

Hampson SE, Skinner TC, Hart J, *et al.* Effects of educational and psychosocial interventions for adolescents with diabetes mellitus: a systematic review. *Health Technol Assess.* 2001; **5**(10): 1–79.

International Diabetes Federation (IDF). *International Standards for Diabetes Education.* Belgium: IDF; 2003.

Joslin EP, Gray H, Root HF. Insulin in hospital and home. *J Metab Res.* 1922; 2: 651–99.

Kaufman FR, Halvorson M, Carpenter S, *et al.* Insulin pump therapy in young children with diabetes. *Diabetes Spectrum.* 2001; **14**(2): 84–9.

Lucas S, Walker R. An overview of diabetes education in the United Kingdom: past, present and future. *Pract Diabetes Int.* 2004; **21**(2): 61–4.

Murphy HR, Rayman G, Skinner TC. Psycho-educational interventions for children and young people with type 1 diabetes. *Diabet Med.* 2006; **23**(9): 935–43.

Murphy HR, Wadham C, Rayman G, *et al.* Approaches to integrating paediatric diabetes care and structured education: experiences from the families, adolescents and Children's Teamwork Study (FACTS). *Diabet Med.* 2007; **24**(11): 1261–8.

National Health Service (NHS) Information Centre. *National Diabetes Paediatric Audit 2008–2009.* Leeds: NHS Information Centre; 2010.

National Institute of Clinical Excellence. *Guidance on the Use of Patient-Education Models for Diabetes: technology appraisal 60.* London: NICE; 2003.

National Institute for Clinical Excellence. *Type 1 Diabetes in Children, Young People and Adults: NICE guideline 15.* London: NICE; 2004.

Swift PG. Diabetes education in children and adolescents. *Pediatr Diabetes.* 2009; **10**(Suppl. 12): 51–7.

Waller H, Eiser C, Knowles J, *et al.* Pilot study of a novel educational programme for 11–16 year olds with type 1 diabetes mellitus: the KICK-OFF course. *Arch Dis Child.* 2008; **93**(11): 927–31.

CHAPTER 10

The role of the diabetes educator

Rebecca Gebert

INTRODUCTION

The role of the diabetes healthcare professional is to help 'replace misunderstanding and fear with knowledge and confidence, contributing to improved compliance with treatment, tighter glycemic control and enhanced psychosocial functioning, contributing in a positive way to their overall health and quality of life' (Aanstoot *et al.*, 2007, p. 26).

The American Association of Diabetes Educators (AADE, n.d.) has defined seven diabetes self-care behaviours that are essential for improved health status and greater quality of life for children, young people and families living with diabetes. These are:

- healthy eating
- being active
- self-monitoring
- taking medication appropriately
- problem-solving
- healthy coping behaviours
- reducing risk behaviours.

The role of structured education programmes as a way of delivering these educational topics has been identified as key (Funnell *et al.*, 2007). The different contributions that members of a multidisciplinary team make in order to provide the knowledge, skills and tools needed to successfully manage diabetes and avoid many of the complications associated with the disease have been discussed in Chapters 7 and 8. However, structured education programmes are often time-limited or only available at specific points in the diabetes journey.

Equally, a referral to a particular team member may only take place when there are significant problems (e.g. to a psychologist when coping strategies have become maladaptive or unhelpful). This contrasts with diabetes education as an ongoing process starting at diagnosis.

This chapter describes the role of the diabetes educator and the part they play in the process of delivering diabetes education on a continuous basis to children, young people and families. The term *diabetes educator* is used here to reflect the way the role is formally defined. However, it is recognised that different team members in a diabetes healthcare team may provide different aspects of the role.

THE HISTORICAL AND EVOLVING ROLE OF THE DIABETES EDUCATOR

Historically, the diabetes nurse specialist provided nursing care and education to people with diabetes (Dunning, 2007). However, the introduction of increasingly complex diabetes regimens (*see* Chapter 1) has created an additional burden on all involved in the support, education and self-care of diabetes (Brink and Moltz, 1997; Funnell *et al.*, 2007). Over the last 2 decades, the emphasis for implementation of intensive diabetes management has been the responsibility of different members of the multidisciplinary team (Brink *et al.*, 2002).

The American Association of Diabetes Educators highlighted the role of the diabetes educator. They noted that, 'incumbent upon diabetes educators [is] . . . to ensure that diabetes self-management education is appropriately tailored and delivered to ensure safe implementation of intensive diabetes management' (Lorenzi *et al.*, 2002, p. 4). The diabetes educator is identified as central within the multidisciplinary diabetes healthcare team in supporting intensive diabetes management, with evidence to support this position coming from the landmark Diabetes Control and Complications Trial/Epidemiology of Diabetes Interventions and Complications (DCCT/EDIC, 2001, 2009; Brink *et al.*, 2002; Lloyd *et al.*, 1993).

Several authors have argued that education is the keystone of diabetes therapy and 'structured self-management education is the key to a successful outcome' (Krone *et al.*, 2009; Swift and ISPAD, 2007, p. 103). In the United States, Canada and Australia, the role of diabetes educator has been well established (Dunning, 2007). The Australian Diabetes Educators Association considers diabetes education to be 'a specific intervention of diabetes treatment, management and care. Diabetes education combines clinical assessment with supporting people with diabetes to gain the knowledge, skills, motivation and confidence [to] . . . effectively manage their condition' (ADEA, n.d.).

Formalised training in specialised diabetes skills, care and management is now offered in specific education programmes developed for healthcare providers (not only nurses) pursuing a career in diabetes care and education (Dunning, 2007). The primary component of diabetes educator training programmes teaches the practitioner how to educate and teach self-care in diabetes and impart diabetes knowledge, skills and management to the person with diabetes (Dunning, 2007; Funnell *et al.*, 2007).

BOX 10.1 The Australian Diabetes Educators Association's definition of diabetes educators

'[H]ealthcare professionals who focus on educating people with and at risk for diabetes and related conditions achieve behavior change goals which, in turn, lead to better clinical outcomes and improved health status. Diabetes educators apply in-depth knowledge and skills in the biological and social sciences, communication, counseling, and education to provide self-management education/self-management training'. (ADEA, n.d.)

The challenge for all members of the paediatric multidisciplinary diabetes healthcare team is the transfer of medical knowledge about the benefits of intensive therapy while emphasising the equally important task of providing support for psychosocial adjustment to dramatically improve long-term quality of life for children and adolescents with diabetes (Brink and Moltz, 1997). Optimal care occurs when there is a united team approach that supports psychosocially informed individualised intensive diabetes management and diabetes care education (Brink *et al.*, 2002; Drotar *et al.*, 2010; Mortensen, 2003; Skinner and Cameron, 2010; Swift *et al.*, 2010).

The diabetes educator offers diabetes self-management education using facilitated learning and creates opportunities to explore health-related behaviours, an opportunity to discuss the demands diabetes imposes on the person and to think about ways to improve adherence and develop motivation (Funnell and Anderson, 2005; Funnell *et al.*, 2007). The role of the diabetes educator is 'complex and constantly evolving' (Dunning, 2007). In countries where it is an established post, it emerges as a crucial element in the multidisciplinary diabetes healthcare team (Dunning, 2007; Lorenzi *et al.*, 2002). It is argued that the central role of a diabetes nurse educator is to provide a link between medical intervention and psychosocial diabetes care (Dunning, 2007; Funnel *et al.*, 2007; Lorenzi *et al.*, 2002). The diabetes educator works with and complements other healthcare providers in the team (Brink *et al.*, 2002).

In many countries, the specific role of diabetes educator has not yet been embraced or established (Dunning, 2007). Many teams consist of a single physician supported by a clinical nurse specialist with little (or no) access to dietetic or psychological support. In these teams, it will fall to the physician and/or the clinical nurse specialist to take on additional roles and become a 'diabetes educator' by default. However, this may be a difficult role to fill. The Diabetes, Attitudes, Wishes and Needs (DAWN) study (Pharmanews.eu, 2008) revealed that 9 out of 10 children and young people lacked adequate support at school, 'only 2 out of 10 healthcare professionals routinely evaluate the psychosocial needs of the young people with diabetes and their families in their care', or gave poor or non-existent age-appropriate education and support to families, and 4 out of 10 caregivers routinely felt overwhelmed by their child's diabetes. Furthermore, these families had received no parent- and family-centred care or support to overcome this stress or 'burnout'. Of significant additional concern, the research showed an overwhelming need for better-facilitated peer support and networking for children, adolescents and caregivers (Pharmanews.eu, 2008; Greene, 2009). Few had been offered the opportunity to meet and talk with other children, adolescents and caregivers living with diabetes (Pharmanews.eu, 2008; Greene, 2009).

Diabetes education and the burden of diabetes

The emphasis on teaching the principle of intensive diabetes self-management rather than acknowledging the importance of adaptive lifestyle choices for intensive control creates an educational dilemma that Skinner and Cameron (2010) call 'subtle definition-creep' (p. 369). The authors suppose when 'pharmaco-technological' processes take precedence, little research or scrutiny is placed on the social implications of 'treatment innovation' on the child, young person or their family (Skinner and Cameron, 2010, p. 370). While there are no marketing efforts or economic incentives to encourage healthcare providers to understand and implement psychosocial healthcare or education into their approach, the system avoids addressing the complex burden diabetes imposes on families (Skinner and Cameron, 2010). Studies have shown that the diabetes burden for children and adolescents is twice that experienced by an adult (e.g. Pharmanews.eu, 2008).

Diabetes self-management education and support must find a balance between intensifying diabetes self-care education and understanding what the wider implications of intensive therapy mean to children, young people and families. Diabetes educators are in a unique position to provide 'unlimited' psychosocial support to help families acclimatise to altering lifestyle choices in order to reach ultimate glycaemic control and 'ensure optimal clinical outcomes' (Skinner and Cameron, 2010, p. 373). Better predictors of glycaemic outcomes for children and young people are associated with innovative 'psychosocial constructs' and a central focus on child-, adolescent- and family-centred interaction, rather than the 'insulin regimen' (Drotar *et al.*, 2010; Funnel and Anderson, 2005; Skinner and Cameron, 2010). The challenge for diabetes self-management education and support is to harness an approach that seeks to understand the 'lay rationalities' of living with diabetes in childhood and adolescent years to better support self-care and in turn glycaemic control (Crossley, 2001; Funnell *et al.*, 2007). Diabetes care has been described as largely a 'self-care' condition, and it is fundamental to remember that children, young people and their families are carrying out self-care independently of a healthcare team for over 90% of the time (Anderson and Patrias, 2007, p. 141).

What is unique about the diabetes educator?

The proximity of the diabetes educator to the family at diagnosis and the ongoing relationship with the family puts them in a position to best understand what diabetes care imposes on the individual and their family (*see* Chapter 2) (Anderson and Patrias, 2007; Nielsen *et al.*, 2007).

Diabetes self-management education must provide safe goals and targets to minimise hypoglycaemia, as well as ensuring adequate psychosocial support and age-specific approaches to intensive diabetes management in childhood (Skinner and Cameron, 2010). The diabetes healthcare team legitimises health behaviours necessary for metabolic control, which include performing blood glucose monitoring and adherence to an insulin regimen. However, increasingly diabetes self-management education and support focuses on self-treatment and facilitating the person to become their own director of 'diabetes health' (Brink *et al.*, 2002). In many situations, the team will seek health behaviour change by re-educating, advising, persuading, warning or just referring them to another healthcare specialist (Rollnick *et al.*, 2008). This approach fails to understand the personal nature or health beliefs about living with diabetes when associated with 'failure' or 'non-adherence' or 'poor glycaemic control', and it prevents valuable insights about the inefficiency of many approaches to diabetes self-management education (*see* also Chapters 8 and 11) (Crossley, 2001; Rollnick *et al.*, 2008; Sawyer *et al.*, 2007; Schiffrin, 2001).

A diabetes educator can empower or facilitate change and address the psychosocial, developmental and risk factors that lead to poorer adherence, community connectedness and mental health outcomes by providing individualised diabetes self-management education and support (Funnell and Anderson, 2005; Funnell *et al.*, 2007). In this way, diabetes educators take out of practice what does not work and start to look for ways of approaching diabetes self-management education and support that can make a difference.

Therefore, the role of diabetes educator will include sharing and collaborating with respect to knowledge, care and approaches with healthcare teams and other healthcare providers, and, most important, with the child, young person or their family. The diabetes educator must use an effective and 'skilful clinical style' in conversations with children and adolescents and their families that are collaborative in order to have the potential to 'make a difference' to health behaviour and to have long-term influence on glycaemic control (Rollnick *et al.*, 2008; Sawyer *et al.*, 2007; Schiffrin, 2001). Motivational interviewing, goal-setting and decision-making have been found to be an effective way to approach positive behaviour change (*see* Chapter 11) (Drotar *et al.*, 2010; Funnel and Anderson, 2005; Rollnick *et al.*, 2008).

The diabetes educator's role centres on providing diabetes education that allows the person to acquire self-care diabetes skills and to change behaviour to promote self-management (Brink *et al.*, 2002; Funnel *et al*, 2007; Soundarya *et al.*, 2004). As mentioned, an expectation of the role is to increase knowledge, updating and assessing self-care skills and supporting changes to self-management. Insight about the impact of such factors as food choices, physical activity, stress/illness, and medication on blood glucose levels can facilitate adjustments to maintain blood glucose levels within an agreed target range. Diabetes education should focus on providing self-care skills and tools in order to support children and young people to learn to manage their diabetes (Brink *et al.*, 2002). However, it is a challenge to ensure that children and young people remember information and remain motivated to keep carrying out these behaviours. Schiffrin (2001) points out that inadequate self-management is the most frequent problem encountered by diabetes healthcare teams, and particularly educators. This is further supported by Drotar *et al.* (2010), who suggest that non-adherence to medical treatment in 'paediatric chronic illness' is at 'rates of 50%', or potentially higher, despite a good level of knowledge about what they should be doing (p. 1).

Assessment and engagement

As discussed in Chapter 7, a cycle of ongoing referrals to different team members in response to declining glycaemic control and poor adherence can often lead to frustration and little progress or change. The role of a diabetes educator is to seek an understanding of the psychosocial functioning of the child, young person or their family in order to create individualised diabetes care that will lead to 'acquisition of new information and the skills necessary to make informed choices about diabetes care' (Brink *et al.*, 2002, p. 2). In the United Kingdom, there are multidisciplinary teams where the physician, a psychologist and a clinical nurse specialist perform this, but this is not currently the norm. The diabetes educator can offer consistent contact with the child or young person and their family to facilitate preventive interventions that allow further developmental progress, family and diabetes-related functioning, and support diabetes health behaviours. This will also support early identification of psychosocial adjustment problems or psychiatric disorders. The diabetes educator can ensure access to a range of appropriate interventions that might include family, psycho-educational, home-based multi-systemic, peer-group or motivational interviewing interventions that can be offered by the relevant professional (*see* Chapter 12).

The diabetes educator's role is to keep detailed documentation about how the child or adolescent presented at diagnosis, who was involved with the diabetes care education, the family structure and the presence of other extended or family members, as well as developments over the life course of the diabetes to assemble insights into family functioning and adaptation, which can then be communicated with the diabetes team (Brink *et al.*, 2002; Schiffrin, 2001). The diabetes educator can explore the psychosocial dimensions of a family and locate this contextual understanding into individualised diabetes care education. A social ecological model places the child in the centre of an interconnecting network that includes family, neighbourhood, educational environment and also their peers (Hoey, 2009). It also seeks to integrate the family's extended community that includes economic, social, cultural, and political influences and beliefs (Hoey, 2009).

The family-centred 'circle of influence', or the 'children's circle tool', developed by the DAWN study team (*see* Figure 10.1), emphasises all interactions that may influence the ability of the child or young person to manage their diabetes and, as a result, influence their metabolic control (Hoey, 2009). The child or young person is identified as central; however, their family network, the educational environment, the healthcare system, their culture and wider community must also be recognised as important by the multidisciplinary team (*see* Chapter 7) (Hoey, 2009).

Diabetes educators can use the 'circles of influence' to identify significant people in the child or young person's life that may be able to contribute to diabetes self-care. These often include a wide array of individuals that are significant in the child or young person's life, like relatives (grandparents), nanny, teachers and school nurses, sports coaches and religious individuals (such as a priest, rabbi or imam). The diabetes educator has the opportunity of time with families, allowing the families to explore and engage in a regular but informal contact, which can lead to sharing of personal experience in the context of the family.

When psychosocial risks are identified, appropriate referrals to social workers or mental health teams can be facilitated (Sawyer *et al.*, 2007). In an ideal situation, these professionals should be embedded within the team, have expertise in diabetes and participate in team meetings to ensure interventions are integrated into the wider support programme (Brink *et al.*, 2002).

The diabetes educator can also assess the learning styles of the child or

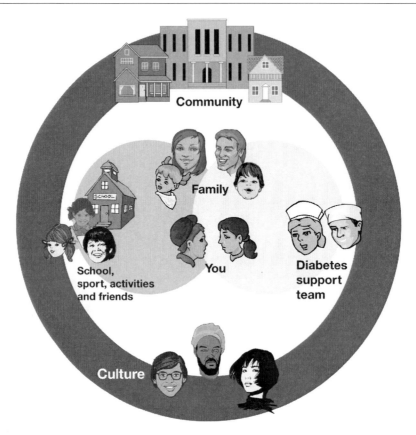

FIGURE 10.1 The children's circle tool

adolescent and their parents, personality traits, and consider the cognitive and developmental level before embarking on diabetes care education (Funnell *et al.*, 2007). This approach requires flexibility and a range of teaching tools to support the educational needs of the child, the young person or the family. The diabetes educator will integrate assessments by different members of the multidisciplinary diabetes team in order to design a learning package based on the child, young person or families' needs.

SPECIFIC DEVELOPMENTAL ISSUES

The partnership between the diabetes educator and children, young people and their family or caregivers is often intense. In teams with a diabetes educator, they are often the first professional in the multidisciplinary team to meet the family as soon as they arrive in the hospital. The first meeting will explain the key aspects of diabetes self-care, including discussions around supporting blood glucose testing and insulin administration. The first experience of self-care is critical. When children, young people or their families have experienced difficulties at the time of diagnosis, ongoing open and honest discussion to explore self-care of blood glucose monitoring and insulin regimen choices can be much harder.

The diabetes educator is in an ideal situation to discuss concerns that can arise at specific developmental stages and consider how best to address these. Diabetes self-management education and support are an ongoing process, and regular consideration of whom else needs to be introduced to the 'circle of interest' leads ongoing review (Funnell and Anderson, 2005; Funnell *et al.*, 2007).

Preschool

For the infant or preschool child, the family is the patient (Aanstoot *et al.*, 2007). The focus should be to help parents and significant others, such as older siblings, grandparents, uncles and aunties, nannies, day-care and kindergarten personnel to understand and manage the diabetes (Aanstoot *et al.*, 2007; Brink *et al.*, 2002). It is important to discuss the impact of the diagnosis and diabetes care on the parent's perception of the additional 'burden' of diabetes care, as this can have an impact on adjustment (*see* Chapter 2). Diabetes self-management education and support is more complicated and difficult to manage for a small child with no written or language skills.

Fear of hypoglycaemia

An often neglected issue for parents is fear of hypoglycaemia. This can be experienced as *I do all the right things, but I still cannot get it right.* The fear of hypoglycaemia drives health beliefs and behaviours that include taking less insulin or eating more as a 'survival' strategy (Halvorson, 2005; Haugstvedt *et al.*, 2010) The parent (or young person) focuses on the everyday risks associated with hypoglycaemia rather than the longer-term consequence of poor control. The view of 'immediacy of risk' to health acts as a barrier or deterrent to aspects of health behaviour as prescribed by the treatment plan (*see* Chapter 3) (Crossley, 2001).

School and socialising

Children and young people with diabetes should have a school action plan designed to support diabetes self-care at school, support participation in activity or sports clubs and ensure successful school trips. School-age children can explore issues by writing stories, drawing pictures or just explaining in their own words what something means to them.

The diabetes educator can act as a liaison between the school and the healthcare team and can identify shared or conflicting priorities for the child and family that might identify additional people to support diabetes care. An example of this could be discussing how to support and plan for school camps or a sleepover at a friend's or a relative's house.

Emotional well-being

The use of neutral and constructive language is important. The diabetes educator can explore the challenges of growth and development and guide exploration of psychosocial demands of the current situation (Anderson, 2007; Halvorson, 2005). The discussion can include worries that the child (or parent) may be experiencing about particular self-care issues or aspects of care may prevent escalation of anxiety and distress (*see* Chapter 3). Important to remember, discuss and explore is frequency, dosing and timing of blood glucose monitoring and insulin administration. Numerous surveys have reported 50% of young people do not monitor or administer according to the recommendations of their treatment team (Patton *et al.*, 2010, p. 365). Linking children through diabetes camps and/or support groups can be helpful for the children as well as giving parents a break from being responsible for diabetes care.

Adolescence

The specific challenges of adolescence are addressed throughout the book (*see* Chapters 4, 6 and 14). The diabetes educator can help in the transition from paediatric to adolescent services, encouraging young people to meet with the healthcare team independently (Court *et al.*, 2008; Surís *et al.*, 2008). Changes in adolescence, such as wanting to sleep in, late nights, poorer food choices, more competitive sport, learning to drive, exams and an increase in risk activities, can all impact on diabetes control and management (Brink *et al.*, 2002; Court, 2008; Skinner and Hampson, 2001). Many health professionals believe for adolescents, 'a psychosocial review of systems is at least as important as the physical exam' (Goldenring and Rosen, 2004, p. 1). A popular and effective tool for interview is the HEADSS psychosocial interview for adolescents (Cohen *et al.*, 1991; Goldenring and Rosen, 2004, p. 1). This interview guide concentrates on core important aspects of adolescent development and comprehensively covers aspects of the 'Home environment, Education and employment, Eating, peer-related Activities, Drugs, Sexuality, Suicidality/depression and Safety from injury and violence' as a conversationally styled psychosocial interview (Goldenring and Rosen, 2004, p. 1). It can be used to cover all aspect of psychosocial influences, burdens, barriers and risks (*see* Part III).

Transition

The diabetes educator is also ideally placed to discuss transition to young adult diabetes services and explore health-related risk behaviours and the issue of complications using decision-making and solution-based approaches, doing so in a positive rather than a frightening or coercive manner (Brink *et al.*, 2002) (*see* Chapter 12). As many adolescents rate their life satisfaction and health perception lower than peers without diabetes, discussions around their life worries, concerns and views on their health can play an important part in decision-making that involves self-care beliefs (Court *et al.*, 2008; Delamater, 2009). The adolescent can be supported to think about how to communicate and negotiate when difficulties arise, build conflict-resolution skills or seek help. Encouraging adolescents to choose follow-up or review by telephone, email, text or other creative ways using information technology may be useful (Court *et al.*, 2008). The diabetes educator must build a 'trusting and motivating relationship' and create an environment for open-ended discussion, engaging in problem-solving and encouraging target-setting, and decisions about treatment options may be discussed and explored from the adolescent's point of view, with the understanding and support of his or her family (Court *et al.*, 2008; Delamater, 2009).

Parents

Social isolation in parents can also be overlooked. The diabetes educator can talk with parents about challenges in getting out and meeting friends and other families. They can discuss what parents could do to discuss their child's diabetes with other people. Linking parents in the early stages with other families or diabetes support groups can allow parents to experience information sharing, parental support and networking. This is often appreciated, as parents have a great sense that the other parent will have empathy and understanding of living with diabetes.

The diabetes educator can also support parents with the transition to greater independence in self-care. Concerns may focus on poor food choices and skipping snacks, not enough recorded blood glucose levels or wanting their adolescent to try a more intensive insulin regimen (Aanstoot, 2007). More serious issues, such as insulin omission or 'forgetfulness', refusal to perform blood glucose levels or fictitious tests being recorded, involvement in 'binge-style' eating or 'insulin purging', may also be reported by parents; these issues need to be taken seriously and should be addressed directly (Aanstoot, 2007). The diabetes educator may be able to explore the underlying issues and concerns for the adolescent and their family and consider a shared approach to managing those issues (DCCT/EDIC, 2001, 2009).

SUMMARY

Diabetes educators are crucial to a multidisciplinary healthcare team, and are predominantly responsible for educating, supporting and exploring with children, young people and their families the realities of living with diabetes.

The diabetes educator's role, while central to providing diabetes self-management education and support, also includes – equally essential – an aptitude for exploring with the child, the young person and their family their 'lived reality' of diabetes self-care management. By the very nature of the individualised and family-oriented education and support provided by diabetes educators, they are able to explore, motivate and encourage behavioural change to lessen the psychosocial demands and associated stress of living a childhood with diabetes and an ongoing transition into adulthood with diabetes.

REFERENCES

Aanstoot H, Anderson BJ, Daneman D, *et al.* Diabetes in children: psychosocial aspects. *Pediatr Diabetes.* 2007; 8(Suppl. 8): 26–31.

American Association of Diabetes Educators (AADE). *AADE7 Self-Care Behaviours Handouts.* Available at: www.diabeteseducator.org/DiabetesEducation/Patient_Resources/AADE7_PatientHandouts.html (accessed 3 August 2010).

Anderson B. Providing support and education to children with diabetes: specific needs, special care. *Diabetes Voice.* 2007; **52**: 37–40.

Anderson RM, Patrias R. Getting out a head: the diabetes concerns assessment form. *Clin Diabetes.* 2007; **25**(4): 141–3.

Australian Diabetes Educators Association (ADEA). *The Diabetes Team.* Available at: www.adea.com.au/main/forhealthprofessionals/thediabetesteam (accessed 3 August 2010).

Brink SJ, Miller M, Moltz KC. Education and multidisciplinary team care concepts for pediatric and adolescent diabetes mellitus. *J Pediatr Endocrinol Metab.* 2002. Available at: www.childrenwithdiabetes.com/download/EaMTCCfPaADM_Brink.pdf (accessed 4 August 2010).

Brink SJ, Moltz K. The message of the DCCT for children and adolescents. *Diabetes Spectrum.* 1997; **10**(4): 259–67.

Cohen E, MacKenzie RD, Yates GL. HEADSS, a psychosocial risk assessment instrument: implications for designing effective intervention programs for runaway youth. *J Adolesc Health.* 1991; **12**(7): 539–44.

Court JM, Cameron FJ, Berg-Kelly K, *et al.* Diabetes in adolescence. *Pediatr Diabetes.* 2008; **9**(3 Pt. 1): 255–62.

Crossley ML. Rethinking psychological approaches towards health promotion. *Psychol Health.* 2001; **16**: 161–77.

Delamater AM. Psychological care of children and adolescents with diabetes. *Pediatr Diabetes.* 2009; **10**(Suppl. 12): 175–84.

Diabetes Control and Complications Trial/Epidemiology of Diabetes Interventions and Complications Research Group (DCCT/EDIC). Beneficial effects of intensive therapy of diabetes during adolescence: outcomes after the conclusion of the Diabetes Control and Complication Trial (DCCT). *J Pediatr.* 2001; **139**(6): 804–12.

Diabetes Control and Complications Trial/Epidemiology of Diabetes Interventions and

Complications (DCCT/EDIC) Research Group. Modern-day clinical course of type 1 diabetes mellitus after 30 years' duration: the diabetes control and complications trial/epidemiology of diabetes interventions and complications and Pittsburgh epidemiology of diabetes complications experience (1983–2005). *Arch Intern Med.* 2009; **169**(14): 1307–16.

Drotar D, Crawford P, Bonner M. Collaborative decision-making and promoting treatment adherence in pediatric chronic illness. *Patient Intelligence.* 2010; **2**: 1–7.

Dunning T. The complex and constantly evolving role of diabetes educators. *Diabetes Voice.* 2007; **52**: 9–11.

Funnell MM, Anderson RM. Patient empowerment. In: Snoek FJ, Skinner TC, editors. *Psychology in Diabetes Care.* 2nd ed. Oxford: John Wiley & Sons; 2005. pp. 97–106.

Funnell MM, Brown TL, Childs BP, *et al.* National standards for diabetes self-management education. *Diabetes Educ.* 2007; **33**(4): 599–614.

Greene A. What healthcare professionals can do: a view from young people with diabetes. *Pediatr Diabetes.* 2009; **10**(Suppl. 13): 50–7.

Goldenring JM, Rosen DS. Getting into adolescent heads: an essential update. *Contemp Pediatr.* 2004; **21**: 64.

Halvorson M. Unique challenges for pediatric patients with diabetes. *Diabetes Spectrum.* 2005; **18**(3): 167–73.

Haugstvedt A, Wentzel-Larsen M, Graue M, *et al.* Fear of hypoglycaemia in mothers and fathers of children with type 1 diabetes is associated with poor glycaemic control and parental emotional distress: a population-based study. *Diabet Med.* 2010; **27**(1): 72–8.

Hoey H. Psychosocial factors are associated with metabolic control in adolescents: research from the Hvidoere study group on childhood diabetes. *Pediatr Diabetes.* 2009; **10**(Suppl. 13): 9–14.

Krone N, Hogler W, Barrett TG. Thoughts on paediatric diabetes care in the UK. *Br J Diabetes Vasc Dis.* 2009; **9**: 259–67.

Lloyd CE, Wing RR, Orchard TJ, *et al.* Psychosocial correlates of glycemic control: the Pittsburgh Epidemiology of Diabetes Complications (EDC) Study. *Diabetes Res Clin Pract.* 1993; **21**(2–3): 187–95.

Lorenzi GM, Delahanty LM, Kramer JR, *et al. Intensive Diabetes Management: implications of the DCCT and UKPDS.* American Association of Diabetes Educators: Position Statement. AADE Board approval 2002: 1–5. Available at: www.diabeteseducator.org/ProfessionalResources/Library/PositionStatements.html (accessed 3 September 2010).

Mortensen HB. *Outcome of Quality Management in Paediatric Diabetes Care: experiences from the Hvidoere Study Group on Childhood Diabetes.* Available at: www.hvidoeregroup.org/public_material/Hvidore%20Booklet%20revised%200303.pdf (accessed 29 November 2011).

Nielsen AO, Lewis D, McEnery C, *et al.* Young people's needs and priorities for improved support and education: a call for action. *Diabetes Voice.* 2007; **52**: 41–2.

Patton SR, Eder S, Schwab J, *et al.* Survey of insulin site rotation in youth with type 1 diabetes mellitus. *J Pediatr Health Care.* 2010; **24**(6): 365–71.

Pharmanews.eu. *Urgent Need for Social and Psychological Support for Young People with Diabetes.* 2008, November. Available at: www.pharmanews.eu/novo-nordisk/46-urgent-need-for-social-and-psychological-support-for-young-people-with-diabetes (accessed 23 August 2011).

Rollnick S, Miller WK, Butler C, editors. *Motivational Interviewing in Healthcare: helping patients change behaviour.* New York, NY: Guilford Press; 2008.

Sawyer SM, Drew S, Yeo M, *et al.* Adolescents with a chronic condition: challenges living, challenges treating. *Lancet.* 2007; **369**(9571): 1481–9.

Schiffrin A. Psychosocial issues in pediatric diabetes. *Curr Diab Rep.* 2001; **1**(1): 33–40.

Skinner TC, Cameron FJ. Improving glycaemic control in children and adolescents: which aspects of therapy really matter? *Diabet Med.* 2010; **27**(4): 369–75.

Skinner TC, Hampson SE. Personal models of diabetes in relation to self-care, well-being, and glycemic control: a prospective study in adolescence. *Diabetes Care.* 2001; **24**(5): 828–33.

Soundarya M, Asha A, Mohan V. Role of a diabetes educator in the management of diabetes. *Int J Diab Dev Countries.* 2004; **24**(3): 65–8.

Surís J, Michaud P, Akré C, *et al.* Health risk behaviors in adolescents with chronic conditions. *Pediatrics.* 2008; **122**(2): e1113–17.

Swift PG, International Society for Pediatric and Adolescent Diabetes (ISPAD). ISPAD clinical practice consensus guidelines 2006–2007: diabetes education. *Pediatr Diabetes.* 2007; **8**: 103–9.

Swift PG, Skinner TC, De Beaufort CE, *et al.* Target setting in intensive insulin management is associated with metabolic control: the Hvidoere childhood diabetes study group centre differences study 2005. *Pediatr Diabetes.* 2010; **11**(4): 271–8.

CHAPTER 11

Motivational interviewing

Sue Channon

INTRODUCTION: WHAT IS MOTIVATIONAL INTERVIEWING?

How often have you sat in consultations with children and young people who are living with diabetes and thought, 'if only they would just . . .'. The end of the sentence might include '. . . do their injections', 'take more readings', 'stop worrying' or simply, 'if only they would just LISTEN'. You will hear this voiced by the parents about their child and you may also at times think it about the parents (just as they are thinking it about you). What all these frustrations have in common is the gap between the 'ideal', as you might see it, and the 'reality' – the gap between knowledge and behaviour, between what we want to do and what we actually do. Managing diabetes is like the management of many other aspects of our behaviour. We may have good intentions to engage in healthy behaviours, to change our lives in a positive direction and make substantial, lasting changes. However, sometimes we don't quite follow through or sometimes we can't maintain it. At the heart of this process is ambivalence. We struggle with conflicting motivations and pressures; the change feels too big, the rewards too distant, the personal or financial costs too high, or maybe it was never our idea to change in the first place.

Motivational interviewing (MI) is an approach that seeks to explore ambivalence and activate motivation for change (Miller and Rollnick, 1991). Rollnick and colleagues (2008) describe three communication styles: (i) 'directing', (ii) 'following' and (iii) 'guiding'. All of these styles have their place within helping relationships. MI has been described as a refined form of guiding, helping the patient consider their own situation and find their own solutions. The aim is to elicit the patient's views and to understand the situation from their perspective, including their goals and values. In this approach there needs to be a spirit of collaboration, in which the expertise of the practitioner plays a part but essentially it is the patient's journey and they decide where to go and how to get there. The practitioner uses his or her knowledge and skills to guide the process, connecting what they know about diabetes with the goals of the patient to facilitate a positive change but always respecting the patient's autonomy, as ultimately it is the patient who decides what to do. Often, paradoxically, it is only by acknowledging that they have every right to make no change that a person may make the first move.

MI in health settings

MI has been gaining ground in adult health services since the early 1980s (Miller, 1983), starting in addictions and then developing in the physical health specialties, particularly in relation to chronic health conditions (Rollnick *et al.*, 2008). The evidence base for MI has grown (Burke *et al.*, 2002; Hettema *et al.*, 2005; Rubak *et al.*, 2005) and the ideas have been refined, both in the context of counselling relationships and in connection to other practitioner–patient relationships, including those of nurse, doctor and dietitian (Arkowitz *et al.*, 2007.) In the last 20 years or so, attention has turned to the potential of MI in the paediatric context and the challenges of using it with families and children at different ages and developmental stages (Erikson *et al.*, 2005; Suarez and Mullins, 2008).

THE EVIDENCE BASE FOR MI IN RELATION TO A PAEDIATRIC POPULATION

A lot of the early work describing MI with young people was focused on specific risk behaviours in relation to drug and alcohol use (Baer and Peterson, 2002). Initial pilot studies identified the potential of MI to reduce risk behaviour, improve attendance and improve outcomes. Larger, more rigorous studies have shown greater harm-reduction behaviours using MI than standard care in relation to alcohol and polysubstance use (Erickson *et al.*, 2005).

In a 2008 review of MI and paediatric health behaviour interventions (Suarez and Mullins, 2008), seven out of nine randomised controlled trials in health-related domains, including diabetes, obesity, reproductive health and dental problems, reported positive findings on the effectiveness of MI compared with the control groups. These demonstrated that it is feasible to use MI with teenagers and parents of younger children in a health-related arena and that MI can also be combined with other approaches and interventions such as dietary advice or cognitive behavioural therapy.

Most randomised controlled trials that have specifically addressed type 1 diabetes relate to the adolescent age group (Winkley *et al.*, 2006). In a non-randomised controlled trial (Knight *et al.*, 2003), MI was combined with a narrative therapy approach. Participants experienced a greater sense of control and improved perceptions of their diabetes compared with the control group, who received usual care. Motivation enhancement therapy is an MI-based approach specifically designed to increase motivation to engage with treatment (Miller and Rollnick, 1991). Viner *et al.* (2003) combined this with cognitive behavioural therapy and systemic and narrative approaches in a non-randomised controlled study. Initial outcomes were very positive, with a significant reduction in HbA_{1c} in the intervention arm (mean reduction of 1.5%) and improvements in self-esteem. At the 7- to 12-month follow-up, there was still some reduction maintained, but the difference between the two groups was no longer significant. In two studies of an individualised MI intervention (Channon *et al.*, 2003, 2007) there was a significant reduction in HbA_{1c} and reduction fears about hypoglycaemia, as well as improvements in quality of life and positive well-being. At 24 months, 1 year after the end of the second larger study intervention, there was still a significant difference in HbA_{1c} and also in some of the quality-of-life measures.

There is preliminary evidence to support the use of MI in paediatric healthcare, including diabetes. There are many issues that need resolving before this can become more firmly established: there are only a handful of studies and a small number of participants with limited work within studies on ensuring treatment fidelity, which is a complex process with a non-manualised, very individual approach. There are measures available to address this (Moyers *et al.*, 2007) that will need to be incorporated if the evidence base is to move forward. MI is a deceptively simple approach: while some of the concepts are straightforward to grasp intellectually, the skilful practice of MI takes time, effort and responsiveness to regular feedback. It is a popular intervention, with a lot of introductory courses available; as such, measurement of treatment fidelity is particularly important to ensure that what is being delivered is actually MI-adherent.

The number of studies of MI in paediatric settings being published has appeared to stall in recent years. One approach has been to integrate MI principles within a 'personal trainer' model, using a non-clinical practitioner to deliver a six-session intervention with teenagers (Nansel *et al.*, 2007). This has shown promising results, with lower HbA_{1c} in the intervention group at 9, 18 and 24 months post-baseline. It was a more effective intervention with older teenagers. These results demonstrate that psychosocial interventions incorporating MI principles delivered by non-clinical practitioners with appropriate levels of training can have a lasting impact that is clinically meaningful. Recent work looking at interventions with adherent-promoting components has demonstrated that multicomponent interventions that target emotional, social or family processes that facilitate diabetes management have a greater impact than those interventions that just target a direct behavioural process (Hood *et al.*, 2010). In the United Kingdom, another response to the scarcity of mental health resources available to deliver MI interventions has been to shift the focus away from individualised support outside clinic time and towards weaving the ideas into the routine consultations with the regular practitioners, taking a population rather than an individual approach (McNamara *et al.*, 2010).

CORE PRINCIPLES OF MI

The style of interaction and the relationship between a practitioner and patient in MI is often referred to as the 'spirit' of MI. It is a collaborative relationship in which the practitioner evokes from the patient their motivations for change and respects their autonomy and right to make their own choices. MI is an individualised approach, delivered without adherence to a manual, but there are some core principles in its application. Where possible, these principles and the key skills that follow will be illustrated with short examples using two scenarios: (i) Laura, a girl who has recently gone up to high school and is struggling not to eat sweets with her friends after school, and (ii) Jessica, a mother whose 8-year-old son has been fairly recently diagnosed.

Empathy

The cornerstone of MI is empathy – understanding someone else's emotional experience and respecting it, and listening to the person in a way that makes them feel that they are accepted and understood. This level of understanding requires very active, careful listening, and *tuning in* to the patient's meaning. The practitioner's responses, both verbal and non-verbal, convey acceptance and a genuine understanding of the patient's position.

BOX 11.1 Illustrating empathy

Laura: It's really hard, my friends all get to eat what they want whenever they want and I don't get anything.

A non-empathic response
Practitioner: Yes, well you have to get on with it, I'm afraid, otherwise your HbA_{1c} is just going to keep going up.

An empathic response
Practitioner: It feels really unfair and it's difficult for you to say no.

This empathic response conveys understanding of the patient's position. It is more likely to make Laura feel understood rather than criticised and is more likely to facilitate a positive relationship, which opens up opportunities for progress.

Resisting the righting reflex

There is often a real risk in consultations of both parties 'sticking to their guns' – maybe the practitioner is providing lots of well-intentioned advice and the patient is responding with, in their view, valid reasons for not following it. The practitioner wants to lead the patient in the right direction and try to put them on a path that will be helpful for their health. This is referred to as the practitioner's 'righting reflex'. However, the patient probably feels in two minds about the behaviour change, otherwise they would have already acted on it. Consequently, these conversations will be full of 'yes ... but' statements, as the patient justifies their behaviour in response to attempts to persuade them to change. This has often been described as *resistance* sited in the patient. However, in MI, resistance is seen as a response within an interaction and it is identified as any language or actions that signal movement away from change. Practitioners need to respond to this resistance by finding a way to 'roll with it', avoiding the confrontation that will make it more likely that the patient will consider making the change.

BOX 11.2 Example of righting reflex

Laura: I've tried not to go with them but I can't, and my mum doesn't help when she nags me about it when I get in.

In response to this, the practitioner could choose a simple reflection.
Practitioner: You've tried hard not to go with them but you haven't been able to yet.

Or, in what is described as a *double-sided reflection*, they may be able to bring in information the patient has given them earlier to balance out the reflection.
Practitioner: You have said that getting this sorted is important, so you have been trying hard, but this approach to it hasn't been helpful.

Sometimes it can be helpful to offer a *simple reflection* so the patient feels heard and to then shift away from the difficult issue to focus on a potentially more productive area.
Practitioner: You are trying really hard but it's not helping at the moment. You were talking earlier about . . .

Some practitioners may feel this is somehow 'ducking' the issue, but it is far more productive to go with the patient where there is the possibility of change and to wait for a more suitable time or find another approach in the future to broach the issue that is triggering the resistance.

Supporting self-efficacy

In the end, it is the patient and their family who introduce changes in their lifestyle, and the practitioner needs to believe in their capacity to change and support them with the process. Practitioners can refer back to past successes, they can focus on the skills the patient can bring to the task and they can reinforce references to intentions to change. Working with children and young people, with ever-changing development, means that there is frequent change and the practitioner can often reference a developmental shift that they have noticed.

BOX 11.3 Supporting self-efficacy

Practitioner: [to Laura] I remember when you started to do your own injections, taking over from your mum, and you then went to Guide camp – that took some doing!

Practitioner: [to Laura] You were able to manage that party really well, planning in advance and thinking with your mum about what you would say if anyone commented or tried to make you eat something you didn't want to . . .

Practitioner: [to Jessica] So, you were thinking that you would be happy to let Ross do more of his own injections over the summer holidays . . .

When you have worked with families over a long period of time, it is often easy to become problem-focused. Making a conscious effort to remember progress and achievements can help boost everyone's belief in the possibility of change. This could be as simple as looking in the diary they bring and discussing the times the results were going well, rather than going immediately to the times the results were not so good.

Exploring discrepancy

The vast majority of us are aware of the gap between our real and our ideal situations in terms of behaviour and health. Most of us would get a 'could do better' report when we consider what we know would be beneficial in areas of our life like diet and exercise. When we become aware of the discrepancy and the inconsistencies between our current behaviour and our values or future ambitions, it can be an uncomfortable feeling, often referred to as dissonance

(Draycott and Dabbs, 1998). The practitioner helps the patient explore the discrepancy and invites them to think about changes they could make to bring their behaviour more in line with their goals and values to reduce the discrepancy.

BOX 11.4 Exploring discrepancy

Practitioner: [to Laura] So, you want to get your HbA$_{1c}$ down because you know it's too high at the moment, but you are finding it hard not to join your friends in the sweet shop after school . . .

Practitioner: [to Jessica] As his mum, you want to be more relaxed about his diabetes so you can get back to enjoying things together, but it's really hard to not check on him all the time.

KEY SKILLS

There are four key skills at the heart of MI, which are known by the acronym OARS:

1. Open questions
2. Affirmations
3. Reflective listening
4. Summarising.

Open questions

Closed questions can be answered with just a 'yes' or 'no'. Open questions aim to elicit information helping the person think in detail about the issue. Open questions usually begin with 'how', 'why' or 'what', and asked in the spirit of respectful curiosity, they can broaden and deepen the conversation.

What happens when you go to the shop with your friends?
How does it feel when you don't test his blood sugars every couple of hours?

Affirmations

It is important for the practitioner to identify strengths; affirmations are the acknowledgements of positive actions and intentions on the part of the patient. They are more specific and often more behaviourally focused than simple praise and are framed within the values of the patient.

You really wanted to get good exam results and you have worked hard. You deserve to be very proud of yourself.
Being a supportive parent is really important to you so you have spent a lot of time with him helping him to adjust.

Reflective listening

Careful listening is a key skill in empathy, and reflective listening enables the practitioner to respond in a way that conveys understanding by repeating or rephrasing what has been said. In more complex reflections, meaning may be inferred or the emotional dimension of what the patient has described is included in the practitioner's response.

BOX 11.5 Reflective listening

Laura: I've tried loads of different things but my diabetes is still rubbish.

Simple reflection
Practitioner: So you have tried loads of things . . .

Rephrase
Practitioner: It seems like you have tried lots of ways to try and improve things.

Complex reflection
Practitioner: It's difficult to find something that makes a difference.

Complex reflection of emotion
Practitioner: Sometimes it's really disheartening when you put all the effort in and it makes no difference.

Summarising

Practitioners using MI will summarise throughout the consultation. Simple summaries help make sure that they understand the patient and they provide a way of linking topics and concepts that the patient has raised. Longer summaries can be used often as a form of 'punctuation' to move from one topic to another, to clarify a goal that's been set or to end the consultation.

BOX 11.6 Summarising

Short summary
Practitioner: [to Laura] So for you at the moment, you would like to reduce your HbA_{1c} partly for your health and partly because it upsets your mum.

Long summary
Practitioner: [to Jessica] Before we go on to think about . . . can I just make sure I've understood? You have talked about how you would like Ross to be more

independent with his diabetes because that will help free him up to do other things, and also because you know that's the way things need to go. You might be thinking about him doing his own injections but the thing that worries you the most is hypos, and so you are keeping a very close eye on his blood sugars and what he is eating.

SPECIFIC STRATEGIES

The following are examples of specific activities that would typically be included in MI-based consultations.

Agenda setting

As with many other task-focused settings, it is important that the people in the consultation share an understanding of what is going to happen and that each participant gets an opportunity to have the issues 'on the table' that they want to discuss. Setting an agenda may involve simply a verbal exchange at the start of the consultation or it may involve writing the items down. Whatever practical route is used to create the agenda, the crucial dimension is that it is a collaborative process, enabling each person to feel that they have a chance to have their say and get what they want from the meeting.

BOX 11.7 Agenda setting

Practitioner: What would it be useful for us to discuss today?

Jessica: I'm worried about how we are going to cope when we go on holiday.

Practitioner: Okay. So, how to manage when you are away . . .. We can have a think about that. Anything else you'd like to cover?

Jessica: Well he isn't doing many tests at the moment.

Practitioner: So holidays and testing. Anything else you want to think about today?

Jessica: No, don't think so . . .

Practitioner: Okay, that's fine. Would it be alright if I also put the move up to high school on the list, as I think it might be helpful to think about that a little.

Asking permission

Asking permission to impart information is an important part of adopting a guiding style. This enhances the patient's sense of autonomy and self-efficacy. It lowers resistance, because the patient is actively seeking the information and has the opportunity to say no. It helps to facilitate the collaborative nature of the relationship, reducing the sense of an expert imposing knowledge and moving towards a shared venture. Some examples have been included in the scenarios above including 'would it be alright if . . .?' and 'can I just make sure . . .?'

> *I was wondering if it would be helpful for you if I mentioned some of the things other parents have found useful?*

Exploring pros and cons

Whatever behaviour is under discussion, it is likely that the patient feels some ambivalence about it, otherwise they would either have dismissed it out of hand or they would have gone ahead and implemented it. Uncertainties can exist across emotional, practical and behavioural domains. Reviewing the advantages and disadvantages of the status quo, and similarly the advantages and disadvantages of the change the patient is considering, will help the practitioner understand his or her position and heighten awareness. This activity, often referred to as 'pros and cons', can help clarify the key factors associated with change.

BOX 11.8 Pros and cons: exploring advantages

Practitioner: We have been talking about whether you are happy to let Ross do his own injections. Would it be okay if we thought about the advantages and disadvantages for you of making that change?

Jessica: Yes, okay.

Practitioner: Perhaps first of all you can think about the advantages of keeping things as they are?

Jessica: Well, we seem to be doing fine and his results are pretty good.

Practitioner: So his control is pretty good. Any other advantages . . .?

Once the patient has finished the list of advantages of staying the same, the conversation would move on to the disadvantages.

BOX 11.9 Pros and cons: exploring disadvantages

Practitioner: [to Jessica] So those are the advantages for you of keeping things as they are. Can we turn now to the disadvantages of keeping things the same? What are the disadvantages do you think of not making the change?

This process would continue until all of the advantages and disadvantages of the *change/no change* positions had been explored, increasing awareness and understanding for all. This may seem like a fairly lengthy process, but it does often highlight previously unknown or unacknowledged issues, as well as further establishing practitioner neutrality about change.

Importance and confidence

When the patient is clearly ambivalent about change, it can be helpful to unpick the reasons for their uncertainty. The concepts of importance, confidence and readiness – and the distinctions between them – are central to this exploration of ambivalence in MI (Rollnick *et al.*, 2008). In this strategy, the patient is asked to put a numerical value between 0 and 10 on how important a change is to them. This can then be followed up with questions such as why it was a '4' rather than a '2', or how it would need to change to become a '5'. This provides a useful, more neutral way of talking about change and the personal factors affecting it. It also helps the practitioner think with the patient about the nature of their ambivalence. For example, if a particular change is scored 6 on importance and 3 on confidence, the discussion will be focused on building confidence. If the scores are reversed, then the personal relevance of change is low, so exploring the advantages and disadvantages of change, or other areas of change, may be the next step.

BOX 11.10 Importance and confidence

Practitioner: So you have been talking about Ross doing his own injections. Can I ask you how important would you say it is to you to make this change? For example, what number would you give it on a scale from 1 to 10, where 1 is not at all important and 10 is vitally important?

Jessica: I would think about a 7.

Practitioner: Right, about a 7. I was wondering, what makes it a 7 rather than a 5 or a 6?

The patient can then describe some of the reasons why it is important to them.

Practitioner: Next, I wonder if I can ask you to think about confidence in making that change. So, on a similar scale from 1 to 10, how confident would you say you are that you can make this change – where 1 is not at all confident and 10 is extremely confident?

Jessica: About a 4.

Practitioner: Okay, about a 4. What would have to happen for you to give that a score of 5?

The patient may then describe reasons why their confidence is low and, with the practitioner, consider how it could be improved. The practitioner can go on to explore the relationship between importance and confidence. In this example, as there is a lower score for confidence than importance, the focus of the work would be on helping the parent build her confidence to make the change.

A typical day

Patients want practitioners to understand the impact diabetes has on their day-to-day life, so understanding their context can help (Beresford and Sloper, 2003). By asking them to take you through a typical day in some detail, in 5–10 minutes, the practitioner can begin to grasp the practical and psychosocial aspects of living with diabetes. This process can generate helpful information about who does what in the family and, with teenagers particularly, it can clarify their levels of independence.

BOX 11.11 A typical day

Practitioner: It is really helpful for me to understand how diabetes affects your day-to-day life. That can be a pretty difficult question to answer in general, so I sometimes find it helps if you take me through a typical day, starting when you get up. Then we can think about the times when things go well, and when they are a struggle, and the things you are doing to manage the diabetes day to day. Would that be okay? . . . So, take me through a day – you choose the day . . .

THE JOURNEY OF CHANGE

Sometimes, particularly when people feel very stuck or a change feels too big, it can be hard to imagine making progress. As part of the understanding of diabetes in the broader context of a person's daily life and also being clear that change is a very personal process, it can be helpful to think about how they usually go about change, not just in relation to their diabetes but also in other areas of their life. Learning new skills is something children and young people are familiar with, but they may not have thought about bringing that experience to bear in relation to their diabetes. Typical examples included in their personal journeys of change will be in learning a new sport or a musical instrument, or in coping with exams. By reflecting on their strengths, previous successes, factors that made a difference, the role of others and so forth, they can begin to see that they have the skills to approach diabetes in the same way. The focus is very much on the 'how' of change rather than the 'why' or the 'what'.

BOX 11.12 The journey of change: building on strengths

Practitioner: I was wondering . . . we all make changes in different ways, and learning to manage diabetes involves learning a lot of new skills. Can you think of something else that you have been learning to do recently – like a new activity or hobby?

Jessica: Well, before Ross was diagnosed I had just started pottery classes.

Practitioner: Great. So tell me about how that was going . . .

Jessica: I went with a friend and it was a bit of a social thing really. I'd managed to make a lot of ashtrays! . . . but I did make one vase that turned out really well.

Practitioner: Lots of trying and then result! Your persistence paid off. Can you think about what type of support was helpful from the teacher?

Jessica: Most of the time I was better by myself, but it was helpful sometimes when she put her hands over mine and made the pot – or whatever – with me.

Practitioner: So from that it sounds like you prefer to be pretty independent and you are good at keeping on trying but sometimes it's good to have practical support. Would you say it's a bit the same with the diabetes . . .?

This exchange helps the practitioner get to know the parent. It normalises the learning process and provides opportunities for affirmation, as well as developing an awareness of what type of support she may want.

WHY MI WITH CHILDREN AND YOUNG PEOPLE?

A review of MI in paediatric health settings concluded that, 'as a supportive, idiographic, brief and autonomy based intervention, MI overlaps with adolescents' competing demands, developing identities and desire to assert independence' (Erickson, 2005, p. 1177).

When considering what will work best for whom and in what circumstances, it is particularly important in paediatric care to consider the developmental stage of the child and family. There needs to be *a goodness of fit* in the language, conceptual complexity, explanations and communication style, both with the child at the heart of the consultation and with the family around them. With its focus on collaboration, support for autonomy and client-led agenda setting, MI converges with the developmental tasks of adolescence as the young person seeks to establish their independent identity and reflect on their core values. It is a time of emotional plasticity, which on the one hand creates the significant oscillations in behaviour that so often frustrate those around them, but on the other hand can also provide such fertile ground to consider options for the future. It is also important to bear in mind that not every adolescent is chomping at the bit to escape parental control, so any intervention also needs to be able to accommodate parents who often play a vital role in supporting their child with the diabetes through adolescence and beyond.

Using MI with younger children is a trickier case to argue, and it is an ongoing debate within the MI field as to what age you can start to use MI. On a simplistic level, they need to be able to consider the relationship between their behaviour and past, present or future health outcomes, such as the impact of what they eat on their blood glucose levels. This will be more complex than understanding the relationship between behaviour and outcomes in more familiar domains, such as making a mess causing their parents to nag them. There is also the issue of age-appropriate levels of autonomy and volition, as clearly the intervention needs to take the family structure and values into account. In the clinical setting, most encounters in diabetes with pre-adolescents will be in the company of parents, so this is unlikely to present much of a dilemma. If using MI with a family including a younger child, there are some adaptations that can be made; at these times, it can be helpful to be even more transparent about the structure of the session and to use 'signposts' throughout, explaining the shifts or strategies so that the child can understand what is happening. Similarly, with OARS it is useful to start very simply so that the child gets used to the method before increasing complexity. Sometimes quieter or younger children do not immediately respond to reflection in terms of it helping them expand what they were saying, but that does not necessarily mean they do not experience reflection in the same way. It may be that there will be a development from a reflection several statements on and it is for the practitioner to be sensitive to the process. Open questions can be difficult for little ones because they find it hard to get the frame of reference and can worry they are going to say something 'wrong'. The frame can be given by giving them 'either/or' choices or extremes or use scaling (0–10) to give them the context. Almost all children love affirmations, but practitioners need to be on the alert for any black-and-white thinking ('so if I am a really good girl, then my sister is really bad'). It is advisable to avoid the use of emotionally loaded or judgemental words such as 'good' and to use instead language that is more descriptive.

SUMMARY

MI is an approach that offers practitioners of all professional persuasions an opportunity to engage with their patients in a collaborative exploration of the complexities of living with diabetes. The core principles and strategies can be adapted for use with children, teenagers and parents, and can, with time, training and practice, be introduced within routine consultations.

It is early days in terms of evidence to support the use of MI in paediatrics, and the methodology is still exploratory in many cases. The 'goodness of fit' between the challenges of adolescence and the key tenets of MI endow the method with high face validity in this clinical context. There are also indications that, as in the field of adult healthcare, MI works well in combination with other approaches. However, 'paediatrics' covers a broad age range with many different developmental stages such that no one method delivered in the same way will fit for all patients. MI is a developing field. The work on MI in groups has undergone a significant change in the last decade and lessons can be learned from individual and group MI that enable further thinking about MI in families – as yet, a largely uncharted territory. The next step for research in MI is the careful delineation of what the active ingredients are for whom, how best to deliver it and in what context.

REFERENCES

Arkowitz H, Westra HA, Miller WR, *et al. Motivational Interviewing in the Treatment of Psychological Problems.* New York, NY: Guilford Press; 2007.

Baer JS, Peterson P. Motivational interviewing with adolescents and young adults. In: Miller WR, Rollnick S, editors. *Motivational Interviewing: preparing people for change.* 2nd ed. London: Guilford Press; 2002. pp. 320–32.

Beresford BA, Sloper P. Chronically ill adolescents' experiences of communicating with doctors: a qualitative study. *J Adolesc Health.* 2003; 33(3): 172–9.

Burke BL, Arkowitz H, Dunn C. The efficacy of motivational interviewing and its adaptations. In: Miller WR, Rollnick S, editors. *Motivational Interviewing: preparing people for change.* 2nd ed. London: Guilford Press; 2002. pp. 7217–50.

Channon SJ, Huws-Thomas MV, Rollnick S, *et al.* A multicenter randomized controlled trial of motivational interviewing in teenagers with diabetes. *Diabetes Care.* 2007; 30(6): 1390–5.

Channon S, Smith VJ, Gregory JW. A pilot study of motivational interviewing in adolescents with diabetes. *Arch Dis Child.* 2003; 88(8): 680–3.

Draycott S, Dabbs A. Cognitive dissonance: 2. A theoretical grounding of motivational interviewing. *Br J Clin Psychol.* 1998; 37(Pt. 3): 355–64.

Erickson SJ, Gerstle M, Feldstein SW. Brief interventions and motivational interviewing with children, adolescents, and their parents in pediatric health care settings: a review. *Arch Pediatr Adolesc Med.* 2005; 159(12): 1173–80.

Hettema J, Steele J, Miller WR. Motivational interviewing. *Annu Rev Clin Psychol.* 2005; 1: 91–111.

Hood KK, Rohan JM, Peterson CM, *et al.* Interventions with adherence-promoting components in pediatric type 1 diabetes: meta-analysis of their impact on glycemic control. *Diabetes Care.* 2010; 33(7): 1658–64.

Knight KM, Bundy C, Morris R, *et al.* The effects of group motivational interviewing and externalizing conversations for adolescents with type-1 diabetes. *Psychol Health Med.* 2003; 8(2): 149–57.

McNamara R, Robling M, Hood K, *et al.* Development and Evaluation of a Psychosocial Intervention for Children and Teenagers Experiencing Diabetes (DEPICTED): a protocol for a cluster randomised controlled trial of the effectiveness of a communication skills training programme for healthcare professionals working with young people with type 1 diabetes. *BMC Health Serv Res.* 2010; **10**: 36–46.

Miller WR. Motivational interviewing with problem drinkers. *Behav Psychother.* 1983; **11**: 147–72.

Miller WR, Rollnick S. *Motivational Interviewing: preparing people to change addictive behaviour.* London: Guilford Press; 1991.

Moyers T, Martin T, Manuel J, *et al. Revised Global Scales: motivational interviewing treatment integrity 3.0 (MITI 3.0).* University of New Mexico, Center on Alcoholism, Substance Abuse and Addictions; 2007. Available at: http://casaa.unm.edu/download/miti3.pdf (accessed 7 October 2011).

Nansel TR, Iannotti RJ, Simons-Morton BG, *et al.* Diabetes personal trainer outcomes: short-term and 1-year outcomes of a diabetes personal trainer intervention among youth with type 1 diabetes. *Diabetes Care.* 2007; **30**(10): 2471–7.

Rollnick S, Miller WR, Butler C. *Motivational Interviewing in Healthcare: helping patients change behaviour.* New York, NY: Guilford Press; 2008.

Rubak S, Sandbaek A, Lauritzen T, *et al.* Motivational interviewing: a systematic review and meta-analysis. *Br J Gen Prac.* 2005; **55**: 305–12.

Suarez M, Mullins S. Motivational interviewing and pediatric health behaviour interventions. *J Dev Behav Pediatr.* 2008; **29**(5): 417–28.

Viner RM, Christie D, Taylor V, *et al.* Motivational/solution-focused intervention improves HbA1c in adolescents with type 1 diabetes: a pilot study. *Diabet Med.* 2003; **20**(9): 739–42.

Winkley K, Ismail K, Landau S, *et al.* Psychological interventions to improve glycaemic control in patients with type 1 diabetes: systematic review and meta-analysis of randomised controlled trials. *BMJ.* 2006; **333**(7558): 65–70.

CHAPTER 12

Psychological approaches to working with families: an example of solution-focused brief therapy

Deborah Christie

INTRODUCTION

A key component of effective chronic care management involving young people and their families or carers is establishing and maintaining the motivation that will enable them to manage the complex juggling act required for effective management of their condition. Adherence to medical treatment has proven to be a very difficult outcome to change, not only in type 1 diabetes (Hampson *et al.*, 2001) but also in paediatric chronic illness in general (Rapoff, 1999). Delamater *et al.* (2001) have argued for the efficacy of a number of psychosocial therapies to improve regimen adherence, glycaemic control, psychosocial functioning and quality of life. However, systematic reviews completed over the last decade have suggested the need for more evidence on psychological intervention effects on treatment adherence and glycaemic control. Educational and psychosocial interventions have been found to have only small to medium beneficial effects on physical and psychosocial outcomes (Hampson *et al.*, 2001; Murphy *et al.*, 2006). Generic programmes that focus on knowledge and skills, psychosocial issues, behaviour and self-management result in modest improvements across a range of outcomes, but improvements are often not sustained, suggesting a need for continuous support delivered as part of the care offered by the diabetes team.

Steed *et al.* (2003) focused on the effect of interventions on psychosocial outcomes, including depression, anxiety, adjustment and quality of life, and found that depression seemed to be particularly improved following psychological interventions, while quality of life improved more following self-management interventions. A recent meta-analysis of nearly 1000 adolescents across 15 randomised control trials of adherence interventions for young people with diabetes found that most effective interventions included multiple components (e.g. emotional, social or family targets) in addition to a specific behavioural goal (Hood *et al.*, 2010). Quantitative and narrative analysis of the evidence suggests that interventions are more likely to be effective if they demonstrate the interrelatedness of the various aspects of diabetes management (Delamater *et al.*, 2009). Specific intervention techniques, including motivational interviewing (*see* Chapter 11), positive reinforcement and behavioural contracts, communication skills training, negotiation of diabetes management goals, coping skills training and collaborative problem-solving skills training have also been found to be effective in improving treatment adherence. Behavioural interventions aimed at diabetes self-management that are multi-faceted, tailored to the individual and provided for 6 months or longer also demonstrate modest effects in improving diabetes-related outcomes (Viner *et al.*, 2003; Whittmore, 2006).

In a systematic review of psycho-educational interventions, Hampson *et al.* (2002) reported that only interventions that involved the family were found to have a significant impact on metabolic control and/or family functioning (Satin *et al.*, 1989). This chapter is focused on the clinical description of systemic approaches that are used in solution-focused and narrative therapy. These systemic, brief therapy approaches are being increasingly adopted in clinical practice, both in the United Kingdom and internationally, and have been found to improve engagement in children, young people and families resistant to more traditional psychological intervention models.

Family-based interventions

Family communication and conflict correlate with adherence to treatment for type 1 diabetes and glycaemic control (Anderson *et al.*, 2002). Because of the complexity of diabetes management and the importance of family involvement and support, most interventions include a family component. However, the quality of family relationships may not be causally related to adherence; therefore, decreasing family conflict and improving parent–child relationships may not result in improved adherence or glycaemic control.

In a review of family interventions, Armour *et al.* (2005) found a positive effect of family interventions in five out of 19 randomised controlled trials and argued that interventions with families of people with diabetes may be effective in improving diabetes-related knowledge and glycaemic control. Further, family therapy incorporating developmentally appropriate, negotiated responsibility has been reported to be effective in improving metabolic control (Satin *et al.*, 1989). Multisystemic therapy, an intensive home and community family intervention, significantly improved adherence to blood glucose testing, improved metabolic control and decreased the number of inpatient admissions (Ellis *et al.*, 2004, 2005; Martin *et al.*, 2009).

Behavioural family systems therapy (BFST) is an approach developed for families of adolescents with clinically significant, conduct-related problems (Robin and Foster, 1989). The components of the intervention include cognitive restructuring of irrational beliefs, structural family interventions that target problematic family characteristics, and family communication and problem-solving. Initial adaptations of BFST-based problem-solving and communication training for children and families with diabetes addressed general developmental issues such as managing curfews and chores and focused less on diabetes treatment–related adherence or management (Wysocki *et al.*, 2000, 2001)

Wysocki and colleagues (2000, 2001) found that BFST enhanced family communication, improved parent–adolescent relationships and reduced behaviour problems and general and diabetes-related family conflict (Harris *et al.*, 2001, 2005, 2009). The effects on psychological adjustment to diabetes and diabetic control depended on the adolescent's age and gender, but overall there was little effect on adjustment to diabetes or diabetic control (Wysocki *et al.*, 2000, 2001).

A revised model (BFST-D) integrated empirically supported intervention strategies focusing on specific behaviours as well as the social context of diabetes treatment–related behaviour.

BOX 12.1 BFST-D components

- Targeting at least two or more diabetes problems
- Behavioural contracting (Wysocki *et al.*, 1989)
- Self-monitoring blood glucose data (Anderson *et al.*, 1989; Delamater *et al.*, 1990)
- Parental simulation of living with diabetes (Satin *et al.*, 1989)
- Involving peers, siblings and teachers, and running sessions in different locations.

BFST-D demonstrated decreased family conflict as well as improvements in regimen adherence, as measured by both parent and child interviews. HbA_{1c} was significantly reduced, particularly among adolescents with poor metabolic control. Change in treatment adherence correlated significantly with change in HbA_{1c} at each follow-up (Wysocki *et al.*, 2006, 2007).

BFST is very resource-intensive. It requires highly skilled, trained family therapy practitioners who are able to travel into the family home and community. Therefore, it is an approach that, while potentially helpful, is unlikely to be something that could be easily incorporated into clinical practice at the current time.

SOLUTION-FOCUSED BRIEF THERAPY APPROACHES IN CLINICAL PRACTICE

Solution-focused brief therapy approaches have the potential to offer diabetes teams a way of communicating with young people with diabetes who may be reluctant to engage with standard psychological approaches and encourage greater self-management (Davis *et al.*, 1999, Viner *et al.*, 2003).

Practitioners of solution-focused brief therapy adopt the view that the client is the expert on their problem and invite them to describe how they want things to be, to focus on what is already working and to notice how small changes are possible (George *et al.*, 1990). The change looked for is in how the client sees the world or in how to do things differently. There is no direct attempt to find the cause of the problem or attempt to take the problem away.

These approaches can be powerful facilitators of change and fit with models of empowerment that are seen as increasingly relevant in the management of long-term chronic illness. When all members of the diabetes team are trained to use these approaches in the clinic consultation, engagement and communication with children, young people and their families increases (Christie, 2008). The approach offers teams and families a collaborative way of thinking about difficulties with injections or finger pricks, managing eating difficulties, thinking about how diabetes gets in the way of family communication and finding ways to manage the effects of sadness or anger associated with living with diabetes.

Appreciative free talk

Engaging children and families in a conversation that allows health professionals to get to know the person outside of the problem invites the family to focus on resources rather than deficits. It highlights areas that can be discussed later on and sets the scene for positive change (George *et al.*, 1990). The initial meeting with family should begin by exploring what the young person enjoys and what they are good at, in order to identify examples of strengths, abilities and resources.

> **BOX 12.2** Appreciative free talk
>
> - *Can I get to know you a bit first?*
> - *What do you enjoy at school?*
> - *What is your favourite lesson/subject?*
> - *What do you like doing when you are not at school?*
> - *What else are you good at?*
> - *What do you and your friends enjoy doing?*
> - *What do you like doing out of school?*

Ideas are then discussed about how these skills from a 'non-problem area' can be transferred to the 'problem area'. Examples of doing well at school may suggest intelligence and an ability to learn; having friends may indicate social skills, loyalty and an ability to listen and to help others; hobbies and other activities can be framed as a commitment to enjoying life. Parents are asked to describe strengths and abilities they are proud of in their child.

Setting a focus

Setting a focus is similar to the agenda-setting described in motivational interviewing (*see* Chapter 11). Parents, children – and other health professionals – may have different ideas about what would make a meeting helpful, so everyone is asked what their 'best hopes' are for the consultation. The intention is to invite people to see themselves as experts in their own situation – the belief is that people know what they need to talk about. Parents may want to talk about doing more blood tests, while young people may want to talk about problems at school. This requires a negotiation about how the time in the consultation will be used.

> **BOX 12.3** Negotiating the focus
>
> - *As you have come all the way here to meet us today, I want to be as helpful as I can be. If this was going to be a helpful meeting, what would be different by the end of our conversation?*
> - *How do you want to use our time together for it to be helpful?*

Responding to 'don't know'

Young people who are struggling with diabetes and who may be at the greatest medical risk are often the most difficult to engage in psychological work and seldom want to talk about diabetes (Riekert and Drotar, 1999). For young people who respond 'don't know' to questions about what they want to get from a meeting, the healthcare professional can ask, 'Whose idea was it that you come along to the appointment today?' and follow this by asking what they think 'they' might want to talk about.

BOX 12.4 Responding to 'don't know'

- *What would be your best guess as to why your mum wanted you to come here?*
- *Are they worried about things you are not particularly worried about?*
- *What is the worry making them do?*
- *What would your mum have to notice you doing for her to not want you to be coming here?*

Young people find it easier to identify what other people think the problem is and they are able to describe the effect that this has on the family. Different people will want different things to be sorted. Parents want children to sort out their 'attitude', be aware of potential late effects, or take responsibility for their own care. The medical team wants them to cope better with their diabetes regimen, do more injections or finger pricks, try to not miss injections or stop eating the 'wrong' food. Children and young people are often able to describe these problems and are aware of what they would have to be doing in order for things to be sorted (Christie, 2008).

Externalising the problem

Rather than seeing a problem as a fixed attribute, externalising is a way to separate the person from the problem. Externalising is part of narrative approaches that invite young people to talk about how they could live their life without being pushed around by the problem (Freedman and Combs, 1996; White, 1988). Thus, the 'diabetic girl' becomes the girl who is 'living with the challenges of diabetes'. Finding a shared language allows the healthcare professional and the young person to think how to challenge the problem together.

Families are used to being asked, 'What seems to be the problem?', and they are expecting to talk about it. They often begin to talk about the problem without being asked, in order for people to hear what they have been struggling with. One way to begin to externalise the problem is by asking questions that invite children and families to characterise the problem as something outside themselves that they can have control over.

BOX 12.5 An introduction to diabetes

- *I know this may sound like a funny question, but could you introduce me to diabetes?*
- *When did it turn up at your house?*
- *Where does it live?*
- *If diabetes were sitting on that chair next to you, how would I recognise it? Is it big or small?*
- *Does it remind you of anything?*

Examples of some answers:

- *Mark (8 years old): It's a big purple monster with syringes for teeth and needles for a tail.*
- *Susan (14 years old): It's a bad-tempered imp – called Charlie.*
- *Jane (15 years old): It's like a big, black cloud that follows me around all the time.*

Characterising the problem in this way invites the children and young people to think about how they find ways to tame the monster, stop Charlie spoiling things for them or how they have found ways to shrink the cloud.

Externalising can also be used with other difficulties. Rather than talking with young people about *being* depressed or aggressive, the aim is to try to characterise 'the sadness' or 'the anger' associated with managing the diabetes. The young person is asked to describe what kind of things 'the problem' gets them to do. It's not unusual to be told that anger makes them skip injections or eat chocolate. The next step is to check if they want things to be different and then to ask how they find ways to put anger in its place.

Stepping into the future

In more traditional approaches where people are invited to think about what steps they are going to take to 'solve the problem', it easy to focus on what will make these steps unachievable. De Shazer (1988) noticed that asking people what they were going to do was an unhelpful question. In contrast, inviting people to describe a 'preferred future' – how they would like things to look, without worrying about the steps they would have to take to get there – enabled significant therapeutic change. This approach was developed empirically by De Shazer and colleagues and invites families to describe the future they want when the problem is no longer around and to say how close they already are to this preferred future, as well as identifying what they would be doing if they were one step closer. De Shazer called this approach 'the miracle question' (De Shazer, 1994).

BOX 12.6 The miracle question

I have a strange, perhaps unusual question, a question that takes some imagination . . . suppose . . . after we finish here, you leave, watch TV, have dinner and so on, go to bed . . . and while you are sleeping a miracle happens . . . and the problems that brought you here – to see me – are solved, just like that! But you were sleeping and so you don't know the miracle has happened. So when you wake up in the morning, how will you go about discovering that this miracle has happened to you? What will you be doing or saying or thinking differently that will give you clues that the miracle has happened?

For a younger child, we might say that something 'magic' happened during the night (as if a fairy waved a magic wand). Selekman (1977) invites families to gaze into a 'crystal ball' and describe what they can see happening in the future. We also invite young people to step into a 'time machine' that we keep in the corner of the room and travel forward into the future, then get out and have a look round while they describe what is happening (Selekman, 1997). De Shazer (1988) emphasised the need to be patient and 'wait for the answer'. The healthcare professional can agree that it is a difficult question, and with slightly younger children they can repeat the last part of the question.

The goal is to get as good a picture of the preferred future as possible, with details and concrete examples of what the child or young person will be doing in the future – without having to think about how they got there. If they say they would be 'feeling' happy, they should be invited to say how they would notice they were happier and what their parents, friends or teachers would notice. The healthcare professional can ask where they would be going, or what would they be doing with friends or with parents, whether they would be arguing less with their parents and what they would notice themselves doing and saying if they had more confidence. We also invite parents to tell us what they think they would notice and ask them what they would notice themselves doing or saying differently.

BOX 12.7 Example of discussion following the miracle question

Jane: I wouldn't have diabetes.

Therapist: So what else would you notice?

Jane: I wouldn't be arguing with Mum about my BMs [blood glucose measurement] . . .

Therapist: What would you be doing that would help you notice that you weren't arguing?

Jane: We'd be having breakfast . . . maybe [laughing].

Therapist: What else?

Jane: I'd be going out with my friends . . . for a sleepover . . . going out shopping.

Therapist: What else would you notice?

Jane: Mum wouldn't be phoning me all the time.

Therapist: What else?

Jane: I'd feel more confident.

Scaling

Having got a clear and detailed picture of the preferred future, the next step invites young people to identify where they are in relation to this preferred future (George *et al.*, 1990). This is used to get a sense of what changes the young person has already made and how far they need to travel. With a younger child, we may draw a line on a piece of paper, point to the two ends and ask them to show us on the line where they are.

> *Let's imagine that if things how you have just described them were a 10 . . . and 0 is the furthest away that you could be from this. How close to 10 are you today?*

Young people rarely say they are at 0. The majority of people scale themselves around 3 when first asked. Scaling creates an opportunity for us to ask how come they have managed to take these steps to the future on their own and hear about what has enabled this to happen.

For example, if someone says they are at 3 we can ask:

> *How come you have already been able to get to a 3 on your own?*

If someone is at a 5, we can ask:

> *How come you are already halfway towards how you want things to be?*

or

What have you been doing to get to a 5? Who has helped you do this?

Answers to these questions enable people to say what they would already be doing at the next step and help them break their goals into small, concrete, manageable and observable steps, which are within their power to achieve. For each answer, we ask for descriptions of what they would be doing, noticing or saying:

- *Where would you like to be?*
- *What would be good enough?*
- *What would a 6 look like? What could I do to help you take one step closer?*
- *What would things look like if you were one step closer to 10?*

Looking for exceptions

Assuming that small change is always possible, the healthcare professional can invite children and families to talk about times when they have been close to the miracle – even if only for a brief moment (*see* Box 12.7). De Shazer (1988) called this 'looking for little pieces of the miracle'. These 'sparkling moments' are exceptions to the problem story and identify abilities that can be harnessed to bring about subsequent steps towards the preferred future.

BOX 12.8 Looking for little pieces of the miracle

- *When, even for an instant, were you in charge of the problem?*
- *What did you do?*
- *What did others notice?*
- *Who wouldn't be surprised you were able to do this?*

Coping

If someone does scale themselves at a 0 (or even a negative number), we can ask coping questions in order to hear how come they haven't given up and are still prepared to come to meet us or hear about what has prevented things from getting worse (*see* Box 12.8).

BOX 12.9 Coping questions

- *What have you done to prevent things being worse?*
- *How did you do that?*
- *In which ways was that helpful?*
- *What do you think you would want to continue doing, to get that to happen more often?*
- *How come you haven't given up?*
- *What has stopped you going below a 0?*
- *How come you managed to do what you did today?*

Pulling things together

The diabetes team often hears stories of previous teams who gave lots of advice where 'nothing worked'. Despite this, it is not unusual for parents to say they want us to tell them how to 'sort out the problem' or they want us to give them advice on how to manage a specific situation. Our goal is to invite families to see themselves as the expert, rather than ourselves being the 'experts' and 'giving advice'. If we ignore these warning signs and fall into the 'must do something to help' trap, invariably the family will say, 'Yes, but . . . we already did that'. Molnar and De Shazer (1987) suggest that summarising conversations using the family's words to describe what they wanted to get from the meeting shows that we have been listening carefully. It is important to validate and acknowledge difficulties that have been discussed. However, we can also summarise resources, strengths, skills and abilities, and we can point out steps already taken towards a preferred future.

This approach also creates opportunities for the healthcare professional to invite young people to look out for times that they take a step closer to the miracle, when they notice the diabetes being less of a 'bully' or less scary and ask if they would be willing to come back and tell us what has made this possible.

Responses of families

These conversations can be a very different experience for families who previously might have felt blamed or criticised for the difficulties they have had managing diabetes. Mothers have often been told they are 'anxious' or 'enmeshed', while youngsters are described as 'non-compliant' or 'manipulative'. Health professionals can feel easily moved by the reaction of families when offering them compliments on their commitment to their son or daughter and their determination in ensuring they get the best care. Parents may become tearful when told what a good job they have done bringing up a smart, articulate and engaging young person (who in previous interactions might have been moody and silent). Young people previously described as non-compliant or manipulative 'grow visibly taller in their chair' when congratulated on their talents and abilities.

SUMMARY

There is still insufficient evidence to recommend adaptation of a particular behavioural or educational approach to address all aspects of barriers to treatment adherence and glycaemic control among children and adolescents with type 1 diabetes.

The marked variation in the influences on and barriers to treatment adherence and improving glycaemic control is difficult to address with a single intervention model. Because long-term patterns of treatment adherence and glycaemic control can be influenced by heterogeneous factors (Rapoff, 1999; Riekert and Drotar, 2000), a one-size-fits-all model of family intervention may not have powerful effects on treatment adherence. For some adolescents and their families, problematic communication and problem-solving may be the primary influences on non-adherence to diabetes treatment. For others, maladaptive patterns of coping and behaviour, such as avoidance or skill deficits in diabetes management, may be the most salient barriers to treatment adherence.

Living with diabetes can be challenging and demanding for families and young people striving to achieve regular developmental goals. The relentless daily demands of a diabetes regimen can easily hijack progress and knock young people and their families off track. While integrated psychological support to paediatric and adolescent clinics remains thin on the ground, it is important to identify different approaches that fit for different families and that can be delivered effectively and within resource-driven constraints. Solution-focused brief therapies and other systemic approaches, like motivational interviewing, are increasingly demonstrating positive outcomes both in research and, most importantly, in the experience of clinicians and the children, young people and families they are working with.

REFERENCES

Anderson BJ, Vangsness L, Connell A, *et al.* Family conflict, adherence and glycemic control in youth with short duration type 1 diabetes. *Diabet Med.* 2002; **19**(8): 635–42.

Anderson BJ, Wolf RM, Burkhart MT, *et al.* Effects of peer group intervention on metabolic control of adolescents with IDDM: randomized outpatient study. *Diabetes Care.* 1989; **12**(3): 179–83.

Armour TA, Norris SL, Jack Jr L, *et al.* The effectiveness of family interventions in people with diabetes mellitus: a systematic review. *Diabet Med.* 2005; **22**(10): 1295–305.

Boardway R, Delamater A, Tomakowsky J, *et al.* Stress management training for adolescents with diabetes. *J Pediatr Psychol.* 1993; **18**(1): 29–45.

Brown SJ, Lieberman DA, Gemeny BA, *et al.* Educational video game for juvenile diabetes: results of a controlled trial. *Inform Health Soc Care.* 1997; **22**(1): 77–89.

Christie D. Dancing with diabetes: brief therapy conversations with children, young people and families living with diabetes. *Eur Diabetes Nurs.* 2008; **5**: 28–32.

Cook S, Herold K, Edidin DV, *et al.* Increasing problem solving in adolescents with type 1 diabetes: the choices diabetes program. *Diabetes Educ.* 2002; **28**: 115–24.

Davis ED, Vander Meer JM, Yarborough PC, *et al.* Using solution-focused therapy strategies in empowerment-based education. *Diabetes Educ.* 1999; **25**(2): 249–7.

De Shazer S. *Clues: investigating solutions in brief therapy.* New York, NY: WW Norton; 1988.

Delamater AM. Psychological care of children and adolescents with diabetes. *Pediatr Diabetes.* 2009; **10**(Suppl. 12): 175–84.

Delamater A, Bubb J, Davis S, *et al.* Randomized prospective study of self management training with newly diagnosed diabetic children. *Diabetes Care.* 1990; **13**(5): 492–8.

Delamater AM, Jacobson AM, Anderson B, *et al.* Psychological therapies in diabetes: report of the Psychological Therapies Working Group. *Diabetes Care.* 2001; **24**(7): 1286–92.

Edge JA, Swift PG, Anderson W, *et al.* Diabetes services in the UK: fourth national survey; are we meeting NSF standards and NICE guidelines? *Arch Dis Child.* 2005; **90**(10): 1005–9.

Ellis D, Frey M, Naar-King S, *et al.* Use of multisystemic therapy to improve regimen adherence among adolescents with type 1 diabetes in chronic poor metabolic control: a randomized controlled trial. *Diabetes Care.* 2005; **28**(7): 1604–10.

Ellis DA, Naar-King S, Frey M, *et al.* Use of multi-systemic therapy to improve regimen adherence among adolescents with type 1 diabetes in poor metabolic control: a pilot investigation. *J Clin Psychol Med Settings.* 2004; **11**: 315–24.

Freedman J, Combs G. *Narrative Therapy: the social construction of preferred realities.* New York, NY: WW Norton; 1996.

George E, Iveson C, Ratner H. *Problem to Solution: brief therapy with individuals and families.* London: BT Press; 1990.

Greco P, Pendley JS, McDonell K, *et al.* A peer group intervention for adolescents with type 1 diabetes and their best friends. *J Pediatr Psychol.* 2001; **26**(8): 485–90.

Grey M, Boland E, Davidson M, *et al.* Short-term effects of coping skills training as adjunct to intensive therapy in adolescents. *Diabetes Care.* 1998; **21**(6): 902–8.

Grey M, Boland EA, Davidson M, *et al.* Coping skills training for youth with diabetes mellitus has long-lasting effects on metabolic control and quality of life. *J Pediatr.* 2000; **137**(1): 107–13.

Hains AA, Davies WH, Parton E, *et al.* A stress management intervention for adolescents with type 1 diabetes. *Diabetes Educ.* 2000; **26**(3): 417–24.

Hampson SE, Skinner TC, Hart J, *et al.* Effects of educational and psychosocial interventions for adolescents with diabetes mellitus: a systematic review. *Health Technol Assess.* 2002; **5**(10): 1–79.

Harris MA, Freeman KA, Beers M. Family therapy for adolescents with poorly controlled diabetes: initial test of clinical significance. *J Pediatr Psychol.* 2009; **34**(10): 1097–107.

Harris MA, Greco P, Wysocki T, *et al.* Family therapy with adolescents with diabetes: a litmus test for clinically meaningful change. *Fam Syst Health.* 2001; **19**(2): 159–68.

Harris MA, Harris BS, Mertlich D. Brief report: in-home family therapy for adolescents with poorly controlled diabetes: failure to maintain benefits at 6-month follow-up. *J Pediatr Psychol.* 2005; **30**(8): 683–8.

Hood K, Rohan J, Peterson C, *et al.* Interventions with adherence-promoting components in pediatric type 1 diabetes: meta-analysis of their impact on glycemic control. *Diabetes Care.* 2010; **33**(7): 1658–64.

Howe CJ, Jawad AF, Tuttle AK, *et al.* Education and telephone case management for children with type 1 diabetes: a randomized controlled trial. *J Pediatr Nurs.* 2005; **20**(2): 83–95.

Howells L, Wilson A, Skinner T, *et al.* A randomized control trial of the effect of negotiated telephone support on glycaemic control in young people with type 1 diabetes. *Diabet Med.* 2002; **19**(8): 643–8.

Karaguzel G, Bircan I, Erisir S, *et al.* Metabolic control and educational status in children with type 1 diabetes: effects of a summer camp and intensive insulin treatment. *Acta Diabetol.* 2005; **42**(4): 156–61.

Kumar VS, Wentzell KJ, Mikkelsen T, *et al.* The DAILY (Daily Automated Intensive Log for Youth) trial: a wireless, portable system to improve adherence and glycemic control in youth with diabetes. *Diabetes Technol Ther.* 2004; **6**(4): 445–53.

Laffel LM, Vangsness L, Connell A, *et al.* Impact of ambulatory, family-focused teamwork intervention on glycemic control in youth with type 1 diabetes. *J Pediatr.* 2003; **142**(4): 409–16.

Martin C, Southall A, Liveley K, *et al.* A multisystemic therapy applied to the assessment and treatment of poorly controlled type-1 diabetes (a case study in the U.K. National Health Service). *Clin Case Stud.* 2009; **8**(5): 366–82.

Misuraca A, Di Gennaro M, Lioniello M, *et al.* Summer camps for diabetic children: an experience in Campania, Italy. *Diabetes Res Clin Pract.* 1996; **32**(1–2): 91–6.

Molnar A, De Shazer S. Solution-focused therapy: toward the identification of therapeutic tasks. *J Marital Fam Ther.* 1987; **13**(4): 349–58.

Mulvaney SA, Rothman RL, Wallston KA, *et al.* An Internet-based program to improve self-management in adolescents with type 1 diabetes. *Diabetes Care.* 2010; **33**(3): 602–4.

Murphy HR, Rayman G, Skinner TC. Psycho-educational interventions for children and young people with type 1 diabetes. *Diabet Med.* 2006; **23**(9): 935–43.

Northam EA, Todd S, Cameron FJ. Interventions to promote optimal health outcomes in children with type 1 diabetes: are they effective? *Diabet Med.* 2005; **23**(2): 113–21.

Rapoff MA, Barnard MU. Compliance with pediatric medical regimens. In: Cramer JA, Spilker B, editors. *Patient Compliance in Medical Practice and Clinical Trials.* New York, NY: Raven Press; 1991. pp. 73–98.

Rapoff MA. *Adherence to Pediatric Medical Regimens.* New York, NY: Kluwer Academic/ Plenum Publishers; 1999.

Riekert KA, Drotar D. Who participates in research on adherence to treatment in insulin-dependent diabetes mellitus? Implications and recommendations for research. *J Pediatr Psychol.* 1999; **24**(3): 253–8.

Riekert KA, Drotar D. Adherence to medical treatment in pediatric chronic illness: Critical issues and unanswered questions. In: Drotar D, editor. *Promoting Adherence to Medical Treatment in Chronic Childhood Illness: concepts, models, and intervention.* Mahwah, NJ: Erlbaum; 2000. pp. 3–32.

Robin AL, Foster SL. *Negotiating Parent-Adolescent Conflict: a behavioral family systems approach.* New York, NY: Guilford Press; 1989.

Satin W, La Greca A, Zigo M, *et al.* Diabetes in adolescence: effects of multifamily group intervention and parent simulation of diabetes. *J Pediatr Psychol.* 1989; **14**(2): 259–75.

Selekman MD. *Solution-Focused Therapy with Children: harnessing family strengths for systemic change.* New York, NY: Guilford Press; 1997.

Snoek FJ, Van Der Ven NCW, Twisk JWR, *et al.* Cognitive behavioural therapy (CBT) compared with blood glucose awareness training (BGAT) in poorly controlled type 1 diabetic patients: long-term effects on HbA1c moderated by depression; a randomized controlled trial. *Diabet Med.* 2008; **25**(11): 1337–42.

Steed L, Cooke D, Newman S. A systematic review of psychological outcomes following education, self-management and psychological interventions in diabetes mellitus. *Patient Educ Couns.* 2003; **51**(1): 5–15.

Svoren B, Butler D, Levine B, *et al.* Reducing acute adverse outcomes in youths with type 1 diabetes: a randomized, controlled trial. *Pediatrics.* 2003; **112**(4): 914–22.

Viner RM, Christie D, Taylor V, *et al.* Motivational/solution-focused intervention improves HbA1c in adolescents with Type 1 diabetes: a pilot study. *Diabet Med.* 2003; **20**(9): 739–42.

White M. *The Externalising of the Problem and the Re-authoring of Lives and Relationships. Selected Papers.* Adelaide: Dulwich Centre Publications; 1988.

Whittmore R. Behavioral interventions for diabetes self-management. *Nurs Clin North Am.* 2006; **41**(4): 641–54.

Wysocki T, Green LB, Huxtable K. Blood glucose monitoring by diabetic adolescents: compliance and metabolic control. *Health Psychol.* 1989; **8**(3): 267–84.

Wysocki T, Harris MA, Greco P, *et al.* Randomized, controlled trial of behavior therapy for families of adolescents with insulin-dependent diabetes mellitus. *J Pediatr Psychol.* 2000; **25**(1): 23–33.

Wysocki T, Greco P, Harris MA, *et al.* Behavior therapy for families of adolescents with diabetes: maintenance of treatment effects. *Diabetes Care.* 2001; **24**(3): 441–6.

Wysocki T, Harris MA, Buckloh LM, *et al.* Effects of behavioral family systems therapy for diabetes on adolescents' family relationships, treatment adherence, and metabolic control. *J Pediatr Psychol.* 2006; **31**(9): 928–38.

Wysocki T, Harris MA, Buckloh LM, *et al.* Randomized trial of behavioural family systems therapy for diabetes: maintenance of effects on diabetes outcomes in adolescents. *Diabetes Care.* 2007; **30**(3): 555–60.

CHAPTER 13

Management of diabetes and eating disorders

Janet Treasure and Katie Ridge

INTRODUCTION

Cases of eating disorders in diabetes present clinicians with a number of interesting challenges for which a working knowledge of both conditions is important. Careful attention to weight, food portions, exercise and glucose monitoring are integral parts of the diabetes regimen. However, aspects of diabetes care may also place patients at risk of the development of eating difficulties. Disordered eating behaviours in patients with diabetes hold considerable medical risks, and collaboration across clinical disciplines in the assessment, diagnosis and treatment of this population is essential.

This chapter will discuss the features of eating disorders and factors that are specific to the co-morbidity of eating disorders in diabetes. Difficulties in detection and diagnosis will be described, as well as guidelines for management, highlighting common factors in treatment as well as areas where treatment diverges.

CLASSIFICATION

In the *Diagnostic and Statistical Manual of Mental Disorders*, fourth edition (DSM-IV) (APA, 2000), three broad categories of eating disorder are delineated: anorexia nervosa, bulimia nervosa and eating disorder not otherwise specified (ED-NOS) – entitled atypical eating disorder in the *International Classification of Diseases*, 10th revision (ICD-10; WHO, 1992). Proposals have been made to amend the categorisation of eating disorders in the DSM-5 and these will be described where appropriate.

Anorexia nervosa is characterised by restriction of food intake relative to energy requirements, resulting in a less than minimally expected weight. Sufferers of anorexia nervosa may experience intense fear of gaining weight, or they may undertake persistent behaviours (e.g. fasting, excessive exercise, vomiting or laxative use) to interfere with weight gain, despite already being underweight. Explicit rule-making about the consumption of food is common.

Bulimia nervosa involves recurrent episodes of binge eating, with the DSM-5 requiring that binges take place once a week for a duration of 3 months for diagnosis. Bingeing is followed by counteractive behaviours, either through the use of laxatives or diuretics (purging bulimia nervosa) or periods of fasting or excessive exercise (non-purging bulimia nervosa). In diabetes, insulin omission is recognised as a purging behaviour. The reduction or omission of insulin doses for weight loss will be discussed in detail.

ED-NOS encompasses variants of other eating disorders which are of clinical significance but do not fit the criteria of anorexia nervosa or bulimia nervosa. The DSM-5 proposes the name of ED-NOS be changed to Feeding and Eating Conditions Not Otherwise Classified and it has been proposed that the additional categories are included as follows: (i) atypical anorexia, where all criteria for anorexia are met but weight is within a normal range; (ii) sub-threshold bulimia nervosa and sub-threshold binge eating disorder (BED); (iii) purging disorder (including insulin omission), where purging occurs in the absence of binge eating; (iv) night eating syndrome; and (v) other feeding or eating condition not otherwise specified.

Although BED is defined as a subcategory of ED-NOS in DSM-IV, it has been proposed that BED be recognised as a distinct disorder in DSM-5. BED is defined as recurrent episodes of binge eating where the individual ingests an amount of food that is larger than most people would eat in a similar period of time, accompanied by a feeling of a loss of control over their food intake. Diagnosis requires that three of five behavioural indicators are experienced alongside binge episodes: (i) very rapid eating; (ii) eating until uncomfortably full; (iii) eating large quantities of food in the absence of hunger; (iv) eating alone due to embarrassment; and (v) the experience of disgust, depression or guilt after a binge period. BED involves the occurrence of binge eating at least once a week every 3 months where a binge is not accompanied by an inappropriate compensatory behaviour.

DIABETES-SPECIFIC PURGING: INSULIN OMISSION

Eating disorders and sub-threshold eating disturbances produce very different consequences for individuals with diabetes. One of the most salient differences between the presentation of an eating disorder alone and the co-morbidity of an eating disorder with insulin-dependent diabetes is the availability of insulin omission as a compensatory behaviour. While individuals with an eating disorder alone undertake behaviours such as excessive exercise, laxative abuse and self-induced vomiting as purging methods, patients with diabetes will more frequently manipulate the diabetes regimen through the deliberate missing of injections or dose manipulation to induce glycosuria. The lack of available insulin prevents glucose passing from the blood into the cells, resulting in the body being forced to rely on breaking down protein and fat deposits, thus enabling excess caloric intake without corresponding weight gain. It is well established that insulin omission is the most common purging method in individuals with diabetes and an eating disorder, with as many as 31% of young females with type 1 diabetes acknowledging having previously reduced their insulin to promote weight loss (Polonksy *et al.*, 1994). Insulin omission has been reported to increase throughout the teenage years (Peveler *et al.*, 2005). A long-term follow-up study investigating insulin omission over time found that individuals with higher levels of specific distress problems with diabetes management and overall psychological distress were more likely to continue endorsing insulin omission 11 years from baseline (Goebel-Fabbri, 2009).

Case study 1: Danni

I was about 17 when I began missing injections to try and lose weight. I got the idea from something a nurse had said when I'd visited the clinic . . . I had lost some weight and the nurse asked me if my sugars had been particularly high over the last while. She explained to me about the effects high sugars can have on weight. So that was how it started.

Unlike my friends, who were experimenting with dieting and, in some cases, bulimia, I felt unable to lose weight by not eating. It would've just brought on a hypo. Likewise, exercise and food reduction just took too long . . . so playing with my insulin levels and allowing high sugars was, for me, the 'ideal' solution.

After about a month of missing injections, it became too uncomfortable and I knew it was wrong. I felt really thirsty, but at the same time water wouldn't fix it. My body felt really tight; my skin felt tight. I felt like my brain was slow and dull. As soon as I started injecting again I could feel my body loosening up.

HOW COMMON ARE EATING DISORDERS IN INDIVIDUALS WITH DIABETES?

Eating disorders in the general population are more common in females, and although symptoms can begin in adulthood, the highest incidence is between 10 and 19 years of age. As a result, studies assessing the co-morbidity of eating disorders with diabetes have focused upon individuals with type 1 diabetes.

In young females in the general population, the prevalence rates of anorexia nervosa, bulimia nervosa and ED-NOS are 0.3%, 1% and 1%–3%, respectively (Grilo, 1995; Hoek and Van Hoeken, 2003; Johnson et al., 2001). Much controversy has surrounded whether the prevalence of eating disorders in people with diabetes is higher than these figures.

Studies of the prevalence of eating disorders in diabetes have yielded varied results. A recent systematic review (Mannucci et al., 2005) of controlled studies suggests a significant elevated prevalence of bulimia nervosa in individuals with type 1 diabetes compared with non-diabetic controls (1.73% vs 0.69%) and no difference in the prevalence rates of anorexia nervosa (0.06% vs 0.27%). A large multisite controlled study suggested that young females with type 1 diabetes were 2.4 times more likely than controls to have an eating disorder, with ED-NOS being the most frequent diagnosis (Jones et al., 2000). BED and night eating syndrome are also suggested as having an increased prevalence in individuals with type 2 diabetes (Allison et al., 2007). However, BED is strongly associated with obesity, a condition that often precedes type 2 diabetes and, therefore, it may be that diabetes develops as a consequence of BED. A study comparing obese diabetic participants with obese non-diabetic participants found no significant differences in BED prevalence between groups (Mannucci et al., 2002), indicating that the suggested elevated prevalence rates of BED in individuals with type 2 diabetes may be associated with higher body mass index as opposed to diabetic status.

Sub-threshold eating difficulties

As a result of the medical consequences of eating difficulties in patients with type 1 diabetes, it is clear that the threshold for 'clinical significance' of disturbed eating behaviours ought to be lower for this group. In a sample of 9- to 14-year-olds, Colton and colleagues (2004) found that although girls with and without type 1 diabetes received similar composite scores on the C9EDE (Children's Eating Disorder Examination) (0.31 diabetic vs 0.26 non-diabetic), girls with diabetes were significantly more likely to engage in two or more disturbed eating behaviours, most commonly a combination of strict dieting with intense and excessive exercise. Peveler et al. (2005) suggest that as many as 25% of young females with type 1 diabetes may develop clinically important disturbances of eating habits and attitudes at some point in their lives. Research has documented similar behaviours in young people with type 2 diabetes, with a study of weight-loss practices revealing those with type 2 are more likely to employ unhealthy methods of weight loss, such as fasting and the use of diet aids, than those with type 1 (Lawrence et al., 2008). Developing an understanding and awareness of the types of sub-threshold eating disturbances typically exhibited by youngsters with diabetes is essential, as early intervention is associated with improved prognosis.

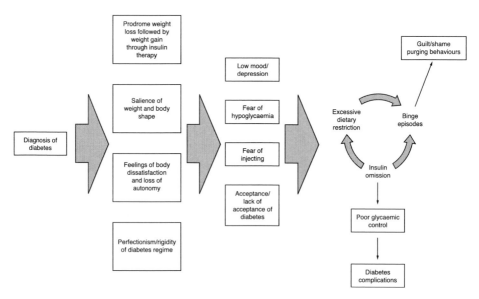

FIGURE 13.1 Diabetes and eating disorders: risk factors

Risk of disordered eating in individuals with diabetes

As already emphasised by the authors of earlier chapters, a diagnosis of diabetes mellitus in childhood challenges a young person at an already difficult developmental stage, where adjustments to diet, lifestyle and healthcare represent huge tasks both for the individual and for their family. While the majority of young people and their families navigate these challenges successfully, a number of characteristics of the diabetes regimen may exacerbate tendencies towards the development of eating disturbances. The behaviours of the young person ought to arouse clinical concern when they are used inappropriately, are employed to excess, interfere with activities of daily living or become a health risk.

Increased attention to weight and shape

Shortly before diabetes is diagnosed, a period of weight loss may occur, which may be experienced as a positive event. The initiation of an insulin regimen brings subsequent unwanted weight gain, thus forging an association in the young person's mind between insulin and their ability to control their weight. Management of diabetes involves increased contact with clinical services that for practical reasons often focus upon the aspects of weight, height and growth, increasing the salience of these physical attributes for the young person. Family members and the clinical team pay attention towards food and nutrition, and there is an expectation upon the young person to monitor what they are eating.

Criticism of weight gain or compliments regarding weight loss from healthcare professionals or family members may reinforce the excessive value of weight control and dieting. Weight and shape concerns as well as lower global and physical appearance–based self-worth have been found to be predictive of disturbed eating behaviours in young females with type 1 diabetes (Olmsted *et al.*, 2008).

Case study 2: Tara

Diagnosed with type 1 diabetes when she was 6 years old, Tara had good control over her blood sugar levels until she was around 13. The hormonal changes of puberty meant that Tara's insulin was not as effective as it had been and this left her with a much harder kind of diabetes to manage at that time. Her parents, not wishing to crowd her, stepped back from her care management just when Tara's diabetes was at its most erratic. Frustrated and with decreased parental supervision, Tara started skipping her insulin. As a result of this, two things happened: Tara's blood sugars rose and she started to lose weight. Many positive comments were made to Tara from both her peers and her family, and Tara accidentally learned that paying less attention to her diabetes and reducing her doses or skipping her insulin altogether was rewarded with positive feedback on her appearance. However, the positive feedback would stop abruptly when she was seen in the diabetes clinic and it was found that her HbA$_{1c}$ had become elevated beyond the target range. Tara is now frequently criticised and blamed by both her healthcare team and her family for this worsening of her diabetes self-management. It is here that disengagement and conflict with her healthcare team begins.

* Vignette adapted from one written and published by Dr Ann Goebel-Fabbri.

A significant psychological impact of the diagnosis

Developing a chronic illness may induce a sense of loss of autonomy and control as well as depressive symptoms (*see* Chapter 2). Excessive weight control practices such as insulin or dietary manipulation could be viewed as a means of regaining control or an attempt to command some sense of responsibility over one's health. Low self-esteem or a negative evaluation of self are both predisposing factors towards disordered eating (Woerwag-Mehta and Treasure, 2008) and have been associated with bulimia nervosa where an individual eats or purges to reduce awareness of the immediate emotional mindset (McManus and Waller, 1995).

Rigidity and perfectionism

Carb-counting, blood glucose testing and the notions of 'good' and 'bad' sugars can exacerbate tendencies towards perfectionism and rigidity, characteristics that have been noted as apparent during childhood after recovery and in the families of individuals who develop eating disorders (Sutander-Pinnock *et al.*, 2003). Cycles of striving for perfection, failing and experiencing guilt or shame can leave an individual feeling 'burnt out' or frustrated with their diabetes (Polonsky, 2002), further affecting their notion of self. The diabetes regimen may also amplify personal traits such as inflexibility or a bias towards focusing excessively upon detail at the expense of seeing the general picture (weak central coherence); these are characteristics that are also seen as common factors in the eating disorder population (Roberts *et al.*, 2007; Lopez *et al.*, 2008).

A different relationship with food

A sense of deprivation associated with dieting as part of diabetes management may lead individuals towards disordered eating behaviours (Rodin *et al.*, 2002). The experience of hypoglycaemia can also entrench maladaptive patterns of eating. Instead of treating a low blood sugar in a measured manner, an individual craving fast-acting carbohydrates may engage in an episode of bingeing, which may induce shame and/or purging (see vignette supplied by Jacqueline Allen, Case study 3, below). Animal models of binge eating describe how addictions to food may emerge. In laboratory rodents where the conditions of binge eating were replicated through food restriction, gastric drainage (an analogue of vomiting), stress and intermittent access to highly palatable food, animals exhibited binge behaviours and also experienced withdrawal symptoms. In individuals with diabetes, binge eating episodes may become part of a vicious cycle, in which negative cognitions and increased psychological distress lead the individual to 'chase' their blood sugars in order to correct them.

Diabetes-specific anxieties

Fears of hypoglycaemia or difficulty injecting insulin may lead young people to omit injections and run sugars high, leading them to 'stumble upon' the role insufficient insulin can play in weight loss. The cycle of insulin omission may be perpetuated in vulnerable individuals.

Case study 3: Ruth

Ruth was 8 when she was diagnosed with type 1 diabetes. Concerned about her health, her parents put their daughter on a strict dietary regimen. Ruth learned there were good foods and bad foods, and quickly becoming preoccupied with her caloric intake and wanting to please her parents. They were delighted that she was so proactive in her own care. Despite her strict food regimen, Ruth, like many other girls with diabetes her age, was slightly heavier than her peers. At the age of 13, she decided to diet. She began by cutting down portions and reducing carbohydrates. Soon, however, Ruth was skipping meals during the day and was rarely eating lunch. At home, her parents noticed that she had become fussier at dinner but were placated by her protestations that it was 'her diabetes' and she knew what was best. Not wanting to suppress Ruth's independence, her parents let her prepare her own dinner and she rarely ate in front of them. Ruth's continued lack of carbohydrate and smaller food intake led to recurrent hypoglycaemia. While hypoglycaemic, Ruth felt unable to control the hunger and began to engage in binge episodes in which she would consume 2000–3000 calories. Following these episodes, she was struck by a sense of having failed at her 'diet' and her diabetes. Dismayed by the high sugar readings she experienced as a result of treating her hypoglycaemia, Ruth started vomiting after each binge episode.

Vignette written by Jacqueline Allan.

MEDICAL RISKS

Disordered eating behaviours in diabetes are associated with impaired glycaemic control (Neumark-Sztainer *et al.*, 2002; Jones *et al.*, 2000) and an earlier-than-expected onset of diabetes-related microvascular complications (Ward *et al.*, 1995; Rydall *et al.*, 1997). Peveler and colleagues (2005) reported a significant relationship between the presence of a probable clinical eating disorder and the occurrence of two or more serious physical complications (including microalbuminuria, proteinuria, retinopathy, neuropathy, dialysis, transplant or death). The use of insulin omission as a purging method in type 1 diabetes may result in recurrent diabetic ketoacidosis (DKA). A study that followed 510 females with diabetes showed that the occurrence of anorexia nervosa with diabetes resulted in a mortality rate of 34.6 per 1000 persons per year, compared with a mortality rate of 2.2 per 1000 persons per year for diabetes alone (Nielsen *et al.*, 2002). National Institute for Health and Clinical Excellence guidelines (2010) highlight the importance of recognising both sub-threshold and clinical cases of eating disorders because of the increased physical risk of this group, and they specify that young persons with type 1 diabetes and poor treatment adherence should be routinely screened for the presence of an eating disorder. As a rule of thumb, poor glycaemic control, repeated episodes of DKA, hypoglycaemia or fluctuations in body weight ought to be important triggers for conversations with young people about their emotional well-being; clinical psychology colleagues should be included at this point in order to understand what additional support may be required.

TABLE 13.1 Diabetes features of eating disorders

Features			
Anorexia nervosa diabetes	Bulimia nervosa diabetes	Binge eating disorder	Eating disorder not otherwise specified
Perfectionism surrounding sugars and excessive testing	Elevated HbA_{1c} Recurrent hospitalisations/ recurrent diabetic ketoacidosis through insulin omission/ purging	Considerable weight gain High insulin requirements High levels of distress/ depression surrounding food intake	Sub-threshold eating difficulties Soon to include purging disorder, including misuse of insulin in the absence of bingeing
Recurrent hypoglycaemia requiring third-party assistance			
Unusual patterns of exercise	Reluctance to inject in front of others		
Insulin omission to prevent hunger	Concurrent psychopathology		
Low mood			
Possible medical concerns regarding purging	Attempts to 'chase' sugars through corrective doses		

SCREENING AND DETECTION

Eating disturbance in young people is a sensitive issue, and detecting it requires careful and considerate questioning. Youngsters may feel ashamed of their behaviours, fearing that they will be criticised. They may be secretive about their eating habits, so establishing rapport and a sense of trust is crucial. The DSM-IV includes insulin omission as a purging method. However, the need to assess the *intention* behind insulin omission is clear, since insulin omission or dose alterations could simply be a method of matching insulin dosage with food intake. Unexplained hyperglycaemia and an elevated HbA_{1c} may involve intake of excess carbohydrates and/or purging through insulin omission, while recurrent hypoglycaemia may be indicative of restrictive eating disturbances, such as excessive dieting or exercise. The discussion of weight and diet ought to become routine between young people with diabetes and members of their clinical team. Box 13.1 details a number of questions that may be helpful in assessing eating habits.

BOX 13.1 Discussing food, weight and insulin omission

- Can you describe how you are feeling about food and diet at the moment?
- What is going well with food?
- What is not going so well?
- How do you feel about your weight and shape?
- People with diabetes often find it difficult to take all of their insulin. How do you find it?
- Thank you for being so honest with me about your insulin habits. Could you tell me a little bit about the times when you don't take your insulin?
- Can you describe any specific reasons why you might not take your insulin?
- Do you notice any disadvantages of not taking your insulin?
- Do you notice any advantages of not taking your insulin?

Psychiatric co-morbidity is common in individuals with eating disorders (Treasure *et al.*, 2009) and screening for coexisting psychopathology is important. Assessment and treatment (where necessary) of depression is particularly pertinent, since as mood improves, the patient may feel more confident about discussing eating behaviours (Ismail, 2008).

Case study 4: Gemma

Gemma was in hospital for diabetic ketoacidosis for the fourth time in 6 months when she confessed to her mother that she had not been taking her insulin in order to lose weight. Diagnosed with type 1 diabetes at the age of 16, Gemma's problems started when she moved away from home to attend university. Insulin therapy had contributed to a significant weight gain and Gemma felt uncomfortable in her new 'fatter' body. Removed from the close supervision of family and resentful of her condition, Gemma stopped paying as much attention to her insulin regimen. Her weight started to fall and she realised that the more food she consumed and the less insulin she took the more weight she could lose. She was initially delighted with this newfound ability to control her weight, receiving positive comments from her new friends and increased male attention.

Gemma soon became terrified of injecting, knowing that it would make her 'fat' and she was binging on high-carb foods to accelerate weight loss. By now, feeling severely ill and barely taking enough long- or short-acting insulin, Gemma realised that she had a major problem. She wanted to talk to a diabetes specialist but because of a missed appointment she had been discharged from her local clinic. At a medication review, Gemma's general practitioner was shocked by her weight loss and referred her urgently to her diabetes centre.

However, Gemma did not attend the appointment for fear of what the doctors would say about her blood sugars. When a concerned friend finally contacted her mother, she demanded that Gemma have a mental health assessment. Gemma was put on a 3-month waiting list. By the time she was seen she had an HbA$_{1c}$ of 17 and had developed retinopathy.

Vignette written by Jacqueline Allan.

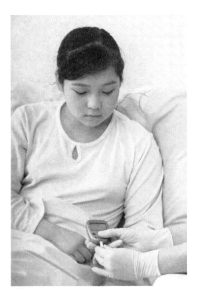

Trying to lose weight by omitting insulin injections is an express route to diabetic ketoacidosis and hospital admission

DIAGNOSTIC TOOLS

The diagnosis of eating disorders in individuals with or without diabetes is a challenge, owing to the considerable overlap across the range of eating disorders. For example, extreme dietary restraint, binge eating and overvalued ideas about weight and shape can be present in all three forms of eating disorder (Treasure *et al.*, 2010). Screening tools such as the eating attitudes test (EAT) or the SCOFF can be used in populations with diabetes. However, caution is needed when utilising screening tools developed for general populations with individuals with diabetes. For example, in the bulimia test revised BULIT-R, the item 'I eat a lot of food even when I'm not hungry' could be over-endorsed among diabetic patients who follow a strict meal plan or who experience and self-treat hypoglycaemia.

Conversely, it is clear that patients who feel additional guilt and shame as a result of non-adherence to the diabetes regimen may be hesitant to describe their eating habits accurately. Kelly *et al.* (2005) make a number of recommendations on how such tools ought to be amended for use with individuals with diabetes, particularly regarding the need to query the intent behind insulin omission, as well as the intent behind any dietary restrictions (i.e. for glycaemic control or weight control). Formal diagnosis should be made by clinical interview with a healthcare professional who has a working knowledge of the diabetes regimen.

A screening tool known as the Diabetes Eating Problem Survey, or DEPS, (Antisdel *et al.*, 2001) has been designed specifically to assess disordered eating in people with diabetes and has been recently validated and revised for paediatric diabetes populations (Markowitz *et al.*, 2010). The tool has demonstrated internal consistency and external validity, takes less than 10 minutes to complete and thus enables the clinician to assess eating behaviour within a regular consultation. Although a tool such as the DEPS cannot provide a conclusive diagnosis, it provides diabetes teams with an accessible method of gauging whether a referral may need to be made to mental health services.

TREATMENT

A common characteristic of eating disturbances is that the individual does not recognise that they have a problem and may indeed be emotionally invested in the behaviours they have been carrying out. Utilising the trans-theoretical model of change (Prochaska and DiClemente, 1983) it can be posited that individuals who are not adhering to elements of their diabetes regimen or engaging in disordered eating behaviours may be in the stage of pre-contemplation, where they see no need to alter their behaviour. As a result, presentation to services is frequently due to coercion by family members or concerned individuals. Even for individuals who recognise that elements of their behaviours have become a health risk and are maladaptive, discussion of eating behaviours and the challenges of diabetes management are issues that may be extremely difficult for the patient to discuss.

As explored in Chapter 11, motivational interviewing is a treatment approach commonly used in eating disorders but also employed in diabetes to empower individuals towards more effective self-care. Adopting a non-confrontational motivational interviewing approach may help to prepare individuals with an eating disorder and diabetes for treatment, where they can discuss their ambivalence about change and may be more willing to engage with services.

Many of the treatment programmes that have been tested in eating disorders have focused on cognitive behavioural therapy (CBT). This approach has garnered considerable support in work with adults, particularly in bulimia nervosa and ED-NOS. Research on the Maudsley model of family therapy has suggested that it is at present the most effective intervention for adolescents with anorexia nervosa and can also be helpful in bulimia nervosa (Keel and Haedt, 2008). However, while many of the approaches to the treatment of an eating disorder *alone* may be considered effective, the treatment of *eating disorder in diabetes* suggests areas where management diverges. For example, treatments for individuals with an eating disorder and diabetes may be enhanced through modifications to include attention to insulin omission, metabolic control, body mass index, diabetes-related dietary restriction, relationships with family and medical caregivers, and feelings about having diabetes.

Modifying eating disorder interventions for patients with diabetes eating disorders

A small study (Peveler *et al.*, 1992) documented the successful use of outpatient CBT and interpersonal therapy for individuals with bulimia nervosa, with the authors highlighting the increased complexity of treating these co-morbidities. A randomised controlled trial assessing the effectiveness of six sessions of psycho-education for females with disordered eating behaviours and their parents successfully reduced dieting, body dissatisfaction and preoccupation with thinness and eating. However, there was no significant change in HbA_{1c} or rates of insulin omission (Olmsted *et al.*, 2002). Takii and colleagues (2003) describe an integrated inpatient programme incorporating eating difficulties and diabetes education that produced marked benefits for patients with type 1 diabetes and bulimia nervosa up until 3 years later, improving glycaemic control and psychological status. This inpatient programme utilised a modified format of CBT where therapists directly intervened to ensure that self-care behaviours were fulfilled. Although inpatient treatment is not routine for patients with bulimia nervosa, this study is an example of how treatments for patients with eating disorders and diabetes may require a different approach.

Regardless of treatment approach, regular physical monitoring of the patient and a collaborative model that empowers the patient towards taking gradual responsibility for their health is crucial. The joint management of cases involving diabetes care teams and child mental health professionals is required, ideally comprising a diabetologist, a diabetes nurse, a dietitian with experience in eating disorders and/or diabetes and a psychologist. In cases of psychiatric co-morbidity, the input of a prescribing physician may be considered, so as to enable possible psychopharmacological intervention. In the United Kingdom, a psychiatrist generally fulfils this function, although specialist nurse prescribers, supervised by psychiatrists, are increasingly taking on this role in multidisciplinary teams. Clinicians from different disciplines may differ on their ideas on first steps, and so collaboration and information exchange is critical if the aim of restoring the patient to their pre-morbid health is going to be achieved.

It is of primary importance to avoid setting difficult or unattainable goals that the patient feels are impossible to achieve, as this may invite feelings of failure or incompetency. It has been suggested that in the short term, focusing excessively upon glycaemic control may in fact be counterproductive (Goebel-Fabbri, 2009; Young-Hyman and Davis, 2010), as such an approach can fail to address psychological difficulties the patient may be experiencing with food. However, flexibility of treatment to suit the individual is important, and for patients who are particularly distressed about their glycaemic control, regulating blood sugars may be their preferred initial target. Ismail (2008) describes how the provision of a continuous subcutaneous insulin infusion pump may alleviate the distress of frequent insulin injections and give the patient confidence in managing everyday activities in preparation for further treatment. Goebel-Fabbri (2009) recommends that an initial focus for treatment could be as small as the patient committing to complete basal insulin doses to prevent future episodes of DKA.

THE ROLE OF THE FAMILY IN EATING DISORDERS AND DIABETES

Although eating disorders were in the past treated on an inpatient basis, clinical guidelines in the United Kingdom now recommend that outpatient treatment should be the preferred initial approach unless a high level of risk is present. This places the primary responsibility for care onto family members, in a situation where parental concerns about the young person's health and safety may already be overwhelming. Parents can experience symptoms of eating disorders as disturbing, frustrating and antisocial. Understandably, hostile confrontations between family members and the sufferer may result, which can paradoxically entrench the undesired behaviours in the individual as opposed to eradicating them. Disturbed family functioning, maternal attachment and maternal eating behaviours have been found to be associated with disturbing eating behaviour in teenagers with type 1 diabetes (Colton *et al.*, 2004; Maharaj *et al.*, 2001).

High levels of expressed emotions displayed by a carer, such as hostility, criticism or overinvolvement, represent natural and indistinctive responses as a result of a desire to care for and protect the sufferer. However, the presence of expressed emotions may further alienate the young person with eating difficulties, forcing them to retreat further into maladaptive behaviours (Treasure *et al.*, 2007a). The protective instincts can be used as a resource for clinicians by inviting parents to take part in the treatment process of eating disorders in diabetes.

The new Maudsley model of collaborative care (Treasure *et al.*, 2007b) offers parents skills in motivational interviewing that have been specifically developed for use in eating disorders. This model of collaborative care involves incorporating the family into the treatment team and recognising carers as a valuable resource for improving the prognosis of the patient. Skills-sharing workshops, where parents are encouraged to reflect upon their emotional reactions to their child's illness and are supported in changing patterns of their behaviour, may be of particular benefit when supporting families with eating disorders in diabetes and have been tested in families of children with type 1 diabetes and suboptimal glycaemic control.

SUMMARY

Eating difficulties that may not be considered noteworthy in the general population are of increased concern in individuals with diabetes. Young people with diabetes have access to a unique purging behaviour in insulin omission, juggling their ability to lose weight rapidly with the risk of poor glycaemic control and long-term complications. A clinician's alertness, not only to eating disorders proper but also to sub-threshold disordered eating behaviours in diabetes, is crucial. Young persons – and particularly young women – with poor glycaemic control should be routinely screened for eating difficulties. Research and clinical experience suggests that levels of 'clinical significance' for eating problems in populations with diabetes should be lowered. Similarly, caution is advised when extrapolating results from screening or diagnostic tools that are not designed for young persons with diabetes. Assessing intent behind insulin omission and dietary practices is vital: careful questioning using a motivational interviewing style may enable clinicians to elicit the patient's beliefs about their eating, weight concerns and diabetes self-care practices. The evidence base for diabetes-specific psychotherapeutic approaches to managing eating problems is still in its infancy, but it is evident that establishing an integrated approach to treatment where endocrinology and psychological services work in tandem is essential. Family interactions in both eating disorders and diabetes are important, and carers are a vital resource for helping patients with their recovery.

ACKNOWLEDGEMENT

We would like to acknowledge the assistance of Jacqueline Allen from Diabetics with Eating Disorders. *See* www.diabeticswitheatingdisorders.org.uk for further information.

REFERENCES

Allison K, Crow S, Reeves R, *et al.* Binge eating disorder and night eating syndrome in adults with type 2 diabetes. *Obesity (Silver Spring)*. 2007; **15**(5): 1287–93.

American Psychiatric Association (APA). *Diagnostic and Statistical Manual of Mental Disorders*. 4th ed., text revision. Washington, DC: APA; 2000.

Antisdel JE, Laffel L, Anderson B. Improved detection of eating problems in women with type 1 diabetes using a newly developed survey. *Diabetes*. 2001; **50**: 47.

Colton P, Olmsted M, Daneman D, *et al.* Disturbed eating behaviours and eating disorders in preteen and early teenage girls with type 1 diabetes: a case-controlled study. *Diabetes Care*. 2004; **27**(7): 1654–9.

Goebel-Fabbri AE. Disturbed eating behaviors and eating disorders in type 1 diabetes: clinical significance and treatment recommendations. *Curr Diab Rep*. 2009; **9**(2): 133–9.

Grilo C. Binge eating disorder. In: Fairburn CG, Brownell KD, editors. *Comprehensive Textbook of Obesity and Eating Disorders*. 2nd ed. New York, NY: Guilford Press; 1995. pp. 178–82.

Hoek H, van Hoeken D. Review of the prevalence and incidence of eating disorders. *Int J Eat Disord*. 2003; **34**(4): 383–96.

Ismail K. Eating disorders and diabetes. *Psychiatry*. 2008; **7**(4): 179–82.

Johnson J, Spitzer R, Williams J. Health problems impairment and illnesses associated with bulimia nervosa and binge eating disorder among primary care and obstetric gynaecology patients. *Psychol Med*. 2001; **31**(8): 1455–66.

Jones J, Lawson M, Daneman D. Eating disorders in adolescent females with and without type 1 diabetes: cross sectional study. *BMJ*. 2000; **320**(7249): 1563–6.

Keel P, Haedt A. Evidence-based psychosocial treatments for eating problems and eating disorders. *J Clin Child Adolesc Psychol*. 2008; **37**(1): 39–61.

Kelly S, Howe C, Hendler J, *et al.* Disordered eating behaviours in youth with type 1 diabetes. *Diabetes Educ*. 2005; **31**(4): 572–83.

Lawrence J, Liese A, Liu L, *et al.* Weight loss practices and weight-related issues among youth with type 1 or type 2 diabetes. *Diabetes Care*. 2008; **31**(12): 2251–7.

Lopez C, Tchanturia K, Stahl D, *et al.* Central coherence in eating disorders: a systematic review. *Psychol Med*. 2008; **38**(10): 1393–404.

Maharaj S, Rodin G, Connolly J, *et al.* Eating problems and the observed quality of mother–daughter interactions among girls with type 1 diabetes. *J Consult Clin Psychol* 2001 December; **69**(6): 950–8.

Mannucci E, Rotella F, Ricca V, *et al.* Eating disorders in patients with type 1 diabetes: a meta-analysis. *J Endocrinol Invest*. 2005; **28**(5): 417–19.

Mannucci E, Tesi F, Ricca V, *et al.* Eating behaviour in obese patients with and without type 2 diabetes mellitus. *Int J Obes Relat Metab Disord*. 2002; **26**(6): 848–53.

Markowitz JT, Butler DA, Volkening LK, *et al.* Brief screening tool for disordered eating in diabetes: internal consistency and external validity in a contemporary sample of pediatric patients with type 1 diabetes. *Diabetes Care*. 2010; **33**(3): 495–500.

McManus F, Waller G. A functional analysis of binge-eating. *Clin Psychol Rev*. 1995; **15**: 845–63.

National Institute for Health and Clinical Excellence. *Type 1 Diabetes in Children, Young People and Adults: NICE guideline 15*. London: NICE; 2010. www.nice.org.uk/guidance/CG15

Neumark-Sztainer D, Patterson J, Mellin A, *et al.* Weight control practices and disordered eating behaviors among adolescent females and males with type 1 diabetes:

associations with sociodemographics, weight concerns, familial factors, and metabolic outcomes. *Diabetes Care.* 2002; **25**(8): 1289–96.

Nielsen S, Emborg C, Mølbak AG. Mortality in concurrent type 1 diabetes and anorexia nervosa. *Diabetes Care.* 2002; **25**(2): 309–12.

Olmsted M, Colton P, Daneman D, *et al.* Prediction of the onset of disturbed eating behaviour in adolescent girls with type 1 diabetes. *Diabetes Care.* 2008; **31**(10): 1978–82.

Olmsted M, Daneman D, Rydall A, *et al.* The effects of psychoeducation on disturbed eating attitudes and behaviour in young women with type 1 diabetes mellitus. *Int J Eat Disord.* 2002; **32**(2): 230–9.

Peveler R, Bryden K, Neil H, *et al.* The relationship of disordered eating habits and attitudes to clinical outcomes in young adult females with type 1 diabetes. *Diabetes Care.* 2005; **28**(1): 84–8.

Peveler R, Fairburn C, Boller I, *et al.* Eating disorders in adolescents with IDDM. *Diabetes Care.* 1992; **32**: 171–6.

Polonsky W. Emotional and quality-of-life aspects of diabetes management. *Curr Diab Rep.* 2002; **2**(2): 153–9.

Polonksy W, Anderson B, Lohrer P, *et al.* Insulin omission in women with IDDM. *Diabetes Care.* 1994; **17**(10): 1178–85.

Prochaska JO, DiClemente CC. Stages and processes of self-change of smoking: toward an integrative model of change. *J Consult Clin Psychol.* 1983; **51**(3): 390–5.

Roberts ME, Tchanturia K, Stahl D, *et al.* A systematic review and meta-analysis of set-shifting ability in eating disorders. *Psychol Med.* 2007; **37**(8): 1075–84.

Rodin G, Olmsted M, Rydall A, *et al.* Eating disorders in young women with type 1 diabetes mellitus. *J Psychosom Res.* 2002; **53**(4): 943–9.

Rydall A, Rodin G, Olmsted M, *et al.* Disordered eating behaviour and microvascular complications in young women with insulin-dependent diabetes mellitus. *N Engl J Med.* 1997; **336**(26): 1849–54.

Sutander-Pinnock K, Blake W, Carter J, *et al.* Perfectionism in anorexia nervosa. *Int J Eat Disor.* 2003; **33**(2): 225–9.

Takii M, Uchigata Y, Komaki G, *et al.* An integrated inpatient therapy for type 1 diabetic females with bulimia nervosa: a 3-year follow-up study. *J Psychosom Res.* 2003; **55**(4): 349–56.

Treasure J, Claudino A, Zucker, N. Eating disorders. *Lancet.* 2010; **375**(9714): 583–93.

Treasure J, Sepulveda A, Whitaker W, *et al.* Collaborative care between professionals and non-professionals in the management of eating disorders: a description of workshops focussed on interpersonal maintaining factors. *Eur Eat Disord Rev.* 2007a; **15**(1): 24–34.

Treasure J, Smith G, Crane, A. *Skills-Based Learning for Caring for a Loved One with an Eating Disorder: the new Maudsley method.* East Sussex: Routledge; 2007b.

Ward A, Troop N, Cachia M, *et al.* Doubly disabled: diabetes in combination with an eating disorder. *Postgrad Med J.* 1995; **71**(839): 546–50.

Woerwag-Mehta S, Treasure J. Causes of anorexia nervosa. *Psychiatry.* 2008; **7**(4): 179–82.

World Health Organization (WHO). *The ICD-10 Classification of Mental and Behavioral Disorders: clinical descriptions and diagnostic guidelines.* Geneva: WHO; 1992.

Young-Hyman D, Davis C. Disordered eating behaviour in individuals with diabetes: importance of context, evaluation, and classification. *Diabetes Care.* 2010; **33**(3): 683–9.

CHAPTER 14

Transition to adult clinics

Helena Gleeson and Janet McDonagh

INTRODUCTION

The term *transition* refers to the process of movement of young people with chronic medical conditions from child- to adult-oriented healthcare systems (Blum *et al.*, 1993). Despite a growing body of research focusing on transition of young people with chronic conditions (Dugueperoux *et al.*, 2008; Frank, 1996; Holmes-Walker *et al.*, 2007; McDonagh *et al.*, 2007; Orr *et al.*, 1996; Robertson *et al.*, 2006; Salmi *et al.*, 1986; Shaw *et al.*, 2007; Steinkamp *et al.*, 2001; Van Walleghem *et al.*, 2008; Vanelli *et al.*, 2004; Zack *et al.*, 2003), evidence to inform design of individual services remains weak (While *et al.*, 2004).

Getting transitional care right for young people with diabetes is essential. Despite strong professional consensus (DoH, 2001, 2005, 2006; NICE, 1994; ISPAD, 2000) on best practice, transition programmes are still not fully integrated into clinical services. A recent national survey of UK diabetes services

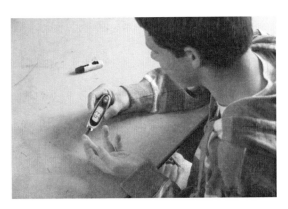

We need to ask ourselves how best to meet the needs of the young person with diabetes

found only 76% had specific local protocols for transition (Gosden *et al.*, 2010). Two years after the introduction of the UK National Service Framework for Diabetes, the challenge of transition services remains (DoH, 2005). Transition is not a stand-alone process, but rather part of the provision of developmentally appropriate healthcare for adolescents and young adults.

With regard to 'the problem of transition', Allen (2009) challenges us to think differently about it: for example, rather than asking how transition should be managed, we might ask ourselves how the needs of young people might best be met.

EVIDENCE TO SUPPORT THE NEED FOR IMPROVING TRANSITION

Transfer between paediatric and adult diabetes services is not always smooth from the young person's perspective. After transfer, 11%–24% of patients with type 1 diabetes fail follow-up in adult clinics (Frank, 1996; Pacaud *et al.*, 1996, 2005). Poor metabolic control, fewer outpatient visits in the year prior to transfer, increased inpatient episodes for diabetes-related illness and not being in post-secondary education are predictors of loss to follow-up in adult services (Frank, 1996; Kipps *et al.*, 2002). Unsurprisingly, this group continues to have poor metabolic control, increased hospitalisation and co-morbidities, both diabetes-related and unrelated (Griffin, 1998; Frank, 1996; Pacaud *et al.*, 1996, 2005). Morbidity associated with transfer of care is also well described in a 5-year Canadian study of 1507 young people with diabetes (Nakhla *et al.*, 2009). Increased inpatient episodes were observed in the 2 years following transfer. The risk of hospitalisation was related to previous inpatient episodes, lower income, female gender and areas with fewer doctors (Nakhla *et al.*, 2009). An Australian study from New South Wales of 239 young adults post-transfer indicated that reduced follow-up, increased use of acute services and poorer metabolic control were associated with follow-up in more regional and less specialised centres (Perry *et al.*, 2010). Nearly 20% of young people with diabetes developed retinopathy or nephropathy when followed longitudinally within 8 years of transfer (Bryden *et al.*, 2001).

The multidimensional nature of adolescent healthcare and transition is often overlooked. Outcomes are mostly limited to medical ones such as metabolic control, complication rates, hospitalisation and/or clinic attendance. However, in a study of young people with cystic fibrosis, even when clinical status remained stable during transfer, educational outcomes were less favourable, with a significant increase in young people not in school or employment (Dugueperoux *et al.*, 2008). A longitudinal study in young people with type 1 diabetes found high rates of obesity, tobacco use and alcohol use within 8 years of transfer (Bryden *et al.*, 2001).

EVIDENCE BASE FOR IMPROVED TRANSITION
Transition models

A recent study commissioned by the National Institute for Health Research (NIHR) Service Delivery and Organisation (SDO) programme to explore transition in diabetes services in the Unite Kingdom identified six different models (Allen *et al.*, 2010; While *et al.*, 2004). Services had been influenced by national guidelines (DoH, 2001, 2005, 2006; ISPAD, 2000; NICE, 1994), clinic attendance, clinical leadership and service user need. Seven dimensions of continuity were identified, adapted from work by Forbes *et al.* (2001).

All services assessed included effective communication between health professionals and services (cross-boundary continuity) and excellent information transfer (informational continuity). They also promoted a therapeutic relationship between the young person and a named health professional appropriate to their needs (relational and longitudinal continuity) (Allen *et al.*, 2010).

Adapting the healthcare system
Importance of relationship with healthcare professionals and continuity of care

Young people and carers have identified that the quality of the relationship with a healthcare professional is important (Allen *et al.*, 2010; Dovey-Pearce *et al.*, 2005; Klostermann *et al.*, 2005; Shaw *et al.*, 2007; Watanabe *et al.*, 2010). Elements important for adolescents in developing a trusting relationship with doctors included fidelity, confidentiality, competency, honesty and a global perspective (Klosterman *et al.*, 2005). This leads to the development of trust and nurtures a non-judgemental approach (Allen *et al.*, 2010). For instance, periods of poor diabetic control as a consequence of the other pressures of adolescence and young adulthood may be understood in the wider context, rather than being attributed to non-compliance (Allen *et al.*, 2010) (*see* Chapter 8).

Provider characteristics are significantly more important determinants of adolescent satisfaction with transition care than physical environment and process issues such as waiting times (Shaw *et al.*, 2007; Watanabe *et al.*, 2010). The most essential aspects of best practice perceived by young people were staff knowledge and staff honesty (Shaw *et al.*, 2007; Watanabe *et al.*, 2010).

Continuity of care is a key issue for young people with diabetes (Dovey-Pearce *et al.*, 2005). In a Delphi study involving young people with arthritis, their parents and professionals, continuity was considered best practice, and feasible, in most hospitals in the United Kingdom (Klostermann *et al.*, 2005). If continuity of healthcare professionals was actively promoted, 77% of young people with diabetes were less likely to be hospitalised following transfer to adult care (Nakhla *et al.*, 2009).

Meeting the adult team

Young people prefer to meet adult team members prior to transfer in diabetes and other chronic conditions (Anthony *et al.*, 2009; Boyle *et al.*, 2001; Kipps *et al.*, 2002; Moons *et al.*, 2009; Scott *et al.*, 2005; Steinkamp *et al.*, 2001; Tuchman *et al.*, 2008). This may be achieved by doctors attending one another's consultations, simultaneously running adolescent and young adult clinics or through organising joint clinics.

Additionally, young people have indicated greater satisfaction if moved from a paediatric to a young adult clinic, rather than directly to an adult clinic; additionally, clinic attendance in the second year has been shown to be higher in young people who met the adult diabetologist prior to transfer (Kipps *et al.*, 2002). However, early introduction to a young adult service can result in a culture shock. Diffusion of responsibility as a result of introducing joint clinics with a multidisciplinary team can result in management discontinuity and may be experienced negatively (Allen *et al.*, 2010). A room full of professionals, some of whom are strangers, can be daunting for anyone – least of all a young person. The alternative of one-to-one consultations may also be equally unappealing!

Roles spanning paediatric and adult services

Transition coordinators can assist young people in navigating the healthcare system by arranging appointments and sending reminders as well as by providing holistic health or psychosocial care (Betz and Redcay, 2005). In the United Kingdom, the diabetes specialist nurse is ideally placed to fulfil this role and is more likely than other providers to demonstrate transition in their practice, offering good management continuity in comparison with the medical team (Allen *et al.*, 2010).

Transition coordinators can have a significant impact on self-care. For example, in a study by Holmes-Walker *et al.* (2007), a transition coordinator reduced admissions and readmissions for diabetic ketoacidosis and reduced length of hospital stay as well as improving metabolic control in 191 young people with diabetes. The Canadian programme called the Maestro Project advocates the role of a 'health navigator' for young people aged 18–30 years. The health navigator serves a primarily administrative role, maintains regular telephone and email contact with patients, arranges drop-in groups, educational events, a website and a monthly newsletter. Implementation of this programme resulted in a 30% reduction in drop-out from diabetes care during a 2-year period, although no short-term health benefits were reported (Van Walleghem *et al.*, 2008).

It is important to recognise the risks in relying on a single individual. Individual relationships can become too close or, conversely, some young people may feel unable to engage with that individual. In addition, departures or absences of the individual may result in complete disruption at an important time. One solution could be to adopt a team approach.

Challenge of continuity of diabetes management and care

A study of users' perceptions of a diabetes clinic for under 25s and their experiences of transferring from paediatric clinic identified clear cultural differences between paediatric and adult teams (Eiser *et al.*, 1993). Paediatric staff placed greater emphasis on family and social life, school and work progress and family relations, whereas adult providers emphasised the risk of long-term complications, the importance of exercise and the need to maintain strict glycaemic control. Eight young people interviewed before and after transfer reported difficulties in transition – in particular, breaking away from established relationships with paediatric service – and they found the medical focus of adult consultations impersonal (Jones *et al.*, 2003). The right to persist with these differing approaches in the management of young people is often justified by 'professional autonomy', arguing young people need to be prepared to adapt to the change in focus of service provision. An alternative view would be that services should change to meet the needs of young people. A real effort should be made to achieve a 'blended' focus, with both teams adopting an adolescent healthcare approach.

One way to blur the boundaries between the culture of care and to achieve continuity of diabetes management, emphasised in the recent NIHR SDO study (Allen *et al.*, 2010) and discussed in the Kennedy report (2010), is clinical leadership and the potential for clinicians gaining dual or specialist qualifications and/or training in this field. Other practical ways of assisting with continuity of diabetes management and care include consensus in management protocols locally and nationally, pre- and post-clinic meetings and formal written communication.

Transfer of information between paediatric and adult services is a concern for young people and their parents (Stabile *et al.*, 2005; Tuchman *et al.*, 2008) and suboptimal information exchange has been reported by several authors (Crosnier and Tubiana-Rufi, 1998; Robertson *et al.*, 2006; Singh *et al.*, 2008). One solution is to provide a written summary for the young person. However, such practices are not universal. In a US study, only 50% of paediatricians provided written transfer summaries for young people with a range of special healthcare needs (Burke *et al.*, 2008). The NIHR SDO study identified that transfer summaries often focus on clinical information, omitting important psychosocial and contextual information (Allen *et al.*, 2010). However, attention to detail of what information is actually transferred is required, as the report of a period of non-adherence at the age of 13 years may no longer be relevant at the age of 18 years and may potentially prejudice the adult team unnecessarily.

Need for information

In a national survey in the United States, only 29% of parents (1411 young people with diabetes) reported prior discussions regarding transfer of care (Lotstein *et al.*, 2009). In a small, co-located team, verbal discussion about the process of transition may be all that is necessary; in a more complex transition service, written information may be necessary (Allen *et al.*, 2010).

Attending to the needs of young people

To attend to the needs of young people, paediatric and adult diabetes services need to adopt a flexible and developmental approach: such an approach emphasises adjustment to the needs of an individual over time and care that adapts to the changing demands of the young person and works to facilitate that change. This enables recognition of the two major frameworks underpinning adolescent healthcare – namely, *development* and *resilience*.

Adolescent development

Transition should start early in adolescence and continue through the mid- and late stages of development, when young people are experimenting with health-risk behaviours and adherence, and when they are testing boundaries. Recent advances in the understanding of adolescent brain development are particularly relevant with respect to adherence and health-risk behaviours (Johnson *et al.*, 2009; Steinberg, 2010). The two main aspects of adolescent brain development are (i) regulation of behaviour and emotion and (ii) perception and evaluation of risk and reward.

Young people with a chronic condition are more likely than their 'healthy peers' to report three or more risk behaviours (Surís *et al.*, 2008). Health-risk behaviours such as substance misuse are associated with non-adherence (Lurie *et al.*, 2000; Stilley *et al.*, 2006). Conversely, the lack of substance use has been reported to be a predictor of successful transfer in a cardiology clinic as defined by attendance at the first adult appointment (Reid *et al.*, 2004) (*see* Chapter 6).

There is a discrepancy between the perception and the evaluation of risk: 10%–39% of young people aged 10–20 years with diabetes reported at least one health-risk behaviour and were aware of the risks but perceived themselves as being less at risk than their healthy peers (Frey *et al.*, 1997).

Brain development is now recognised to continue into the early twenties (Johnson *et al.*, 2009; Steinberg, 2010). The concept of 'emerging adulthood' (Arnett, 2000) notes that whereas identity development is a key milestone in adolescent development, identity exploration is a milestone in emerging adult development (Luyckx *et al.*, 2008).

Young people with diabetes were found to have lower scores on identity exploration in breadth and depth than controls, raising the possibility that young people in this age group perceive fewer opportunities to explore identity issues, owing to illness. In this study, identity development was found to be linked to illness-specific coping and outcomes (Luyckx *et al.*, 2008).

Resilience

Resilience is the capacity of the individual to resist or 'bounce back' in spite of significant stress or adversity (Olsson *et al.*, 2003). Adoption of a resilience framework ensures that as well as the traditional consideration of risk factors, we also consider the protective factors at play, such as the resources available to an individual young person (both intrinsic and extrinsic), their competencies, talents and skills. Murphey *et al.* (2004) reported that the number of 'assets' with respect to school and voluntary work (e.g. talking with parents about school, representation in school decision-making, participation in youth programmes, volunteering in the community) were directly related to health-promoting behaviours and were inversely related to engagement in risk behaviours (Murphey *et al.*, 2004).

One means of assessing resilience (as well as risk) is by using a psychosocial screening tool such as HEADSS (Goldenring and Rosen, 2004). Asking sensitive questions may have potential benefits. Discussion of sensitive issues in a primary care setting was associated with significant benefits. Young people had a more positive perception of the provider and were more likely to have their worries eased, to be allowed to make decisions about treatment and to report taking responsibility for treatment (Brown and Wissow, 2009).

STRUCTURED TRANSITION PROGRAMMES AND INDIVIDUALISED TRANSITION PLANNING

Although recommended, only 50% of clinics surveyed reported a structured transition programme (de Beaufort *et al.*, 2010). Adolescents participating in programmes are more likely to establish care in the adult healthcare system (Tuchman *et al.*, 2008) and may have better clinical outcomes (Cadario *et al.*, 2009; Holmes-Walker *et al.*, 2007). In the evaluation of a transition care programme in rheumatology, self-advocacy skills such as self-medication and seeing professionals independently of parents were reported to predict health-related quality of life (McDonagh *et al.*, 2007).

Individualised transition planning as a collaborative process designed by the young person, the family and their healthcare team is essential. Individualised transition planning is a key component of transitional care, but this has yet to be universally adopted (Hilderson *et al.*, 2009; Lam *et al.*, 2005; Lotstein *et al.*, 2005; McLaughlin *et al.*, 2008; Robertson *et al.*, 2006). The development of written transition plans in diabetes can outline strategies for progressive development of diabetes-related knowledge, disease-management strategies, and self-management skills, as well as addressing psychosocial aspects of growing up with diabetes. They can also help identify educational and vocational goals. Skills that can be nurtured include those of communication, negotiation, goal-setting, problem-solving, decision-making, self-management, information-seeking and disclosure. Transition plans set clear goals for patients and providers (Weissberg-Benchell *et al.*, 2007).

The timing of the initiation of the transition process is important. Most guidance documents advocate a start to transition planning in early adolescence. In a rheumatology study, greater improvements were observed when planning started at age 11 (McDonagh *et al.*, 2006), when young people are already anticipating and/or experiencing change as they move from primary to secondary school.[1] An early start to planning is called for by young people themselves in several studies (Stabile *et al.*, 2005; Tuchman *et al.*, 2008). In contrast, 96% of paediatricians stated that transition should start later than recommended (i.e. within 1 year of the proposed transfer) (Burke *et al.*, 2008). In a recent international survey, 90% of diabetologists recommended that transition planning begin at least 1 year prior to transfer (de Beaufort *et al.*, 2010).

Educational programmes are emerging as an important way to improve patient empowerment in their diabetes care in adulthood, and some programmes are now being trialled with adolescents and young people. In a critical review of diabetes-specific literature, it emerged that educational programmes that were part of a structured transition programme were associated with a measurable outcome of successful transition (Nakhla *et al.*, 2008). Educational programmes in young people with diabetes have been shown to build self-management skills in diabetes and to improve glycaemic control and increase knowledge (Nakhla *et al.*, 2008). However, adequate knowledge does not ensure adequate control (Wysocki *et al.*, 1992). Education programmes accounting for literacy and numeracy have been shown to improve self-efficacy and diabetes control in adult patients (Cavanaugh *et al.*, 2009; Wolff *et al.*, 2009). Developmentally appropriate educational materials and programmes should be developed further and evaluated in young people (Nakhla *et al.*, 2008; Weissberg-Benchell *et al.*, 2007).

Young people with diabetes have also expressed a need for education about the wider aspects of growing up with diabetes, including stress management,

---

1 In the UK education system, most schools are organised into primary schools (up to 11 years) and secondary schools, 11–18 years.

financial matters, sexual development and pregnancy, alcohol and drug use, new developments in diabetes research and healthy cooking (Scott *et al.*, 2005). Counselling and education on the risks associated with alcohol, tobacco and drug use as they relate to diabetes and for sexual and reproductive health form an essential part of any education programme during transition (Mellinger, 2003; Scott *et al.*, 2005).

Residential weekend programmes designed for young people with diabetes, to increase independence through peer support, education and friendship-building, may also have a role. Such programmes have received positive feedback and may facilitate transition, although formal evaluation is lacking (Cuttell *et al.*, 2005).

Checklists are considered integral to individualised transition planning, a feature frequently absent in specialty clinical settings (Hilderson *et al.*, 2009; Lam *et al.*, 2005; McLaughlin *et al.*, 2008; Robertson *et al.*, 2006; Scal *et al.*, 2009). They help identify young people at risk, promote and facilitate opportunities for increasing self-management and track individual young people through the process of transition. From the young person's perspective, it emphasises that it is 'okay to ask' about issues other than disease-specific issues such as substance use, sexual health and so on.

'Readiness' has been recognised as a good predictor for successful transfer for some time (Cappelli *et al.*, 1989; Fredericks *et al.*, 2010; McPherson *et al.*, 2009; Van Staa *et al.*, 2011; Wiener *et al.*, 2007; Williams *et al.*, 2010). Sawicki *et al.* (2011) has recently published preliminary validation data of the Transition Readiness Assessment Questionnaire, which appears useful both to assess transition readiness and to guide educational interventions by providers to support transition. Tools are also being designed for specific conditions, such as the Rotterdam Transition Profile for young adults with cerebral palsy and normal intelligence (Donkervoort *et al.*, 2009). Such tools will potentially be very useful in transition planning from both a clinical and a research perspective.

Young person–friendly service

Paediatric and adult diabetes teams should attempt to provide a service that is developmentally appropriate. A set of quality criteria for this has been defined by the Department of Health called 'You're Welcome' (DoH, 2007), which recommends opportunities to be seen alone, clinics with other young people and the use of methods of communication preferred by young people.

Opportunity for young people to be seen independently has been reported to considered best practice and feasible in the majority of UK clinics by young people with juvenile idiopathic arthritis, their parents and a range of healthcare professionals involved in their care. This was observed as a baseline predictor of improvement in health-related quality of life in young people with juvenile idiopathic arthritis (McDonagh *et al.*, 2007), and as a determinant of successful transfer as defined by attendance at the first adult clinic appointment in cardiology (Reid *et al.*, 2004). Forty-eight per cent of the total variance in transition readiness in adolescents with chronic conditions was explained by perceived self-efficacy in skills for independent hospital visits, independence during consultations and attitude towards transition (Van Staa *et al.*, 2011). Young people also prefer age-banded clinics. However, the number of services adopting this approach in the United Kingdom has fallen from 71% to 44%. It has been emphasised that timing of these clinics should fit in with school and college (Dovey-Pearce *et al.*, 2005; Scott *et al.*, 2005).

Young people have expressed an interest in communication via email or text (Dovey-Pearce *et al.*, 2005; Scott *et al.*, 2005). These methods should reduce concern expressed about decreased contact after transfer to adult services (Tuchman *et al.*, 2008).

Recently, an Internet-based problem-solving tool for adolescents with type 1 diabetes was shown to increase self-management skills by using a combination of multimedia presentations, social networking and email (Mulvaney *et al.*, 2010a, 2010b). The development of user-friendly websites, newsletters and social networking links may also enhance education and awareness of community resources (Weissberg-Benchell *et al.*, 2007).

The online My Health Passport has been used as a novel means of assessing knowledge in young people with chronic conditions (Benchimol *et al.*, 2010), as well as a means of information transfer (Wolfstadt *et al.*, 2010). Web-based discussion forums and social networking enhance peer interaction among adolescents with diabetes (Scott *et al.*, 2005).

TRANSITION AND PARENTS

Research specifically addressing parental aspects of transition is limited, other than the evidence of need in a range of chronic conditions (Geenen *et al.*, 2003; Geerts *et al.*, 2008; Durst *et al.*, 2001; Moons *et al.*, 2009). This includes reports of greater needs than those experienced by the young people themselves (Geerts *et al.*, 2008; Moons *et al.*, 2009). Furthermore, a third of healthcare professionals reported parental difficulties during transition and these professionals perceived parental and family factors as influences of successful transition.

As children make the transition from childhood to adulthood, parents go from parenting a dependent child to parenting an interdependent adult. Getting the balance right is challenging for parents of any teenager, let alone those living with the added challenge of chronic illness and/or disability. A major aspect for the parent of a young person with diabetes is the gradual move from primary responsibility for health management to enabling the young person to self-care. The changing roles with respect to diabetes management during adolescence have been considered extensively in the literature (Dashiff *et al.*, 2008a, 2008b; Schilling *et al.*, 2006).

Studies across several countries indicate that maternal support, conflict, control, involvement and emotional expression are important parent–adolescent communication concepts linked to diabetes outcomes in adolescents (Dashiff *et al.*, 2008a). In a study of young people with congenital heart disease, parents who took total responsibility were less likely to support independence in their adolescent children, who in turn were more likely to be unsure of their diagnosis and less likely to answer for themselves (Clarizia *et al.*, 2009). Parental overprotection has been reported as a key challenge by adolescents with cystic fibrosis post-lung transplant (Durst *et al.*, 2001). In contrast, underprotective parenting has been reported to be associated with non-adherence in another transplant population (Lurie *et al.*, 2000). The major themes in parent–child interactions regarding diabetes management at this age are frustration, fear, normalising, trusting and discounting (Ivey *et al.*, 2009). Ideally, the parent moves from providing all the care to *managing*, as the young person begins to participate in care provision (Kieckhefer and Trahms, 2000). As they become more skilled, the young person takes the role of manager and the parent the *supervisor*; eventually, when competent, the young person becomes their own supervisor, with their parent acting as the *consultant* when problems arise. The recent NIHR SDO study identified the involvement of parents in the transition process as key in supporting management continuity (Allen *et al.*, 2010). During this process, discrepancies regarding the 'right age' and perceived importance of transition issues are likely to arise between health professionals and parents (Geenen *et al.*, 2003) and these need to be sensitively negotiated. The role of the health professional must be that of an extra-parental adult and never as a surrogate parent (Woods and Neinstein, 2008). Transition planning for parents similar to that for the young person has been employed by some researchers and has been found to be useful (McDonagh *et al.*, 2006).

Family dynamics change considerably in adolescence, with young people becoming increasingly emotionally autonomous from parents and wanting to spend more time away from home. The challenge to healthcare providers is advocating for the young person while remaining inclusive of the parents. Understanding the dynamics of individual families, including the predominant parenting style, is vital. Parents have suggested that continuity of professionals and the active involvement of young people during consultations to build trust would help them to gradually withdraw from their primary role in triadic consultations. This would also provide time for their own needs to be met with respect to parenting an adolescent with a chronic illness and/or disability. If parents are to be seen alone, it is important to do this carefully and sensitively during early and mid-adolescence in particular, so as not to lose the trust of the young person. Such service provision has obvious implications for resource allocation in terms of clinic space and time, in addition to staffing levels – particularly for those practitioners not working within a multidisciplinary team.

WORKFORCE COMPETENCY

A workforce competent in adolescent healthcare is integral to the provision of a successful transition service (Kennedy and Sawyer, 2008). Staff trained in adolescent healthcare were considered best practice by an expert panel that included young people and their parents and professionals; however, adequate provision was considered only feasible in a few UK hospitals. A frequently reported barrier to delivery of transition and adolescent healthcare is lack of training (Dieppe et al., 2008; McDonagh et al., 2007).

A preliminary study examining the effect of communication skills in paediatric diabetes services found that although healthcare professionals (doctors, nurses and dietitians) perceived that communication skills to address psychosocial issues were more important than medical issues, confidence in their ability to do so was significantly lower (Hambly et al., 2009). This is similar to other reports from paediatric practices, with a lack of psychosocial assessment documented in 62% of case notes for inpatients aged between 13 and 18 years in a major Australian children's hospital (Yeo et al., 2005), and suboptimal in paediatric rheumatology case notes (Robertson et al., 2006).

Surís et al. (2009) highlighted the need for adolescent training in a study of adult physicians looking after young people with chronic conditions. At least a third of physicians did not discuss sensitive issues, including 73.5% who did not discuss sexual health and 57.8% who did not discuss emotional well-being. Furthermore, only 46% of adult physicians saw such young people independently of their parents – a core component of young person–friendly health services.

Continuity in health personnel has already been commented on and is reported as a key factor for young people with diabetes (Dovey-Pearce et al., 2005), as well as for other chronic conditions. Young people have reported that it takes at least four to five visits before they trust a particular doctor (Klostermann et al., 2005). Training within adolescent clinics brings with it challenges, in that young people may experience an erosion of trust if strangers (e.g. students, trainees) are present during their consultation. Young people say the presence of other healthcare professionals, particularly medical students, significantly inhibits communication with doctors, and limited duration and frequency of contact with the same doctor can impair communication (Beresford and Sloper, 2003).

Training in adolescent health has been associated with sustainable, large improvements in knowledge, skill and self-perceived competency (Sanci *et al.*, 2000, 2005), with higher rates of desired clinical practices such as confidentiality, health screening (Britto *et al.*, 2000; Lustig *et al.*, 2001; Middleman *et al.*, 1995), a higher number of adolescents seen (Key *et al.*, 1995) and a greater tendency to engage in continuing education in adolescent health (Key *et al.*, 1995; Sanci *et al.*, 2005). Part III of this book includes web-based training resources in adolescent healthcare that are useful in both paediatric and adult settings.

SUMMARY

Type 1 diabetes is a long-term condition requiring continuous self-management throughout life. Transition is a key period of time in healthcare for any young person diagnosed with diabetes in childhood. Despite a strong professional consensus on best practice informed by a growing body of research, transition programmes are still not fully integrated into clinical services. To try to address the difficulty of translating research into practice, there is a plea for change in the culture of paediatric and adult services. Transition should be seen as an integral part of adolescent healthcare and there should be a focus on making health services more young person–friendly. To support this, healthcare professionals in paediatric and adult diabetes teams need to gain the necessary knowledge, skills and attitudes to work effectively with young people and their families during transition.

REFERENCES

Allen D, Cohen D, Robling M, *et al. The Transition from Paediatric to Adult Diabetes Services: what works, for whom and in what circumstances? Final Report.* NIHR Service Delivery and Organisation programme; 2010.

Allen D, Gregory J. The transition from children's to adult diabetes services: understanding the 'problem'. *Diabet Med.* 2009; 26(2): 162–6.

Anthony SJ, Martin K, Drabble A, *et al.* Perceptions of transitional care needs and experiences in pediatric heart transplant recipients. *Am J Transplant.* 2009; 9(3): 614–19.

Arnett JJ. Emerging adulthood: a theory of development from the late teens through the twenties. *Am Psychol.* 2000; **55**(5): 469–80.

Benchimol EI, Walters TD, Kaufman M, *et al.* Assessment of knowledge in adolescents with inflammatory bowel disease using a novel transition tool. *Inflamm Bowel Dis.* Epub 2010 Nov 5.

Beresford BA, Sloper P. Chronically ill adolescents' experiences of communicating with doctors: a qualitative study. *J Adolesc Health.* 2003; 33(3): 172–9.

Betz CL, Redcay G. Dimensions of the transition service coordinator role. *J Spec Pediatr Nurs.* 2005; **10**(2): 49–59.

Blum RW, Garell D, Hodgman CH, *et al.* Transition from child-centered to adult health-care systems for adolescents with chronic conditions: a position paper of the Society for Adolescent Medicine. *J Adolesc Health.* 1993; **14**(17): 570–6.

Boyle MP, Farukhi Z, Nosky ML. Strategies for improving transition to adult cystic fibrosis care, based on patient and parent views. *Pediatr Pulmonol.* 2001; **32**(6): 428–36.

Britto MT, Rosenthal SL, Taylor J, *et al.* Improving rheumatologists' screening for alcohol use and sexual activity. *Arch Pediatr Adolesc Med.* 2000; **154**(5): 478–83.

Brown JD, Wissow LS. Discussion of sensitive health topics with youth during primary care visits: relationship to youth perceptions of care. *J Adolesc Health.* 2009; **44**(1): 48–54.

Bryden KS, Peveler RC, Stein A, *et al.* Clinical and psychological course of diabetes from adolescence to young adulthood: a longitudinal cohort study. *Diabetes Care.* 2001; **24**(9): 1536–40.

Burke R, Spoerri M, Price A, *et al.* Survey of primary care pediatricians on the transition and transfer of adolescents to adult health care. *Clin Pediatr (Phila).* 2008; **47**(4): 347–54.

Cadario F, Prodam F, Bellone S, *et al.* Transition process of patients with type 1 diabetes (T1DM) from paediatric to the adult health care service: a hospital-based approach. *Clin Endocrinol (Oxf).* 2009; **71**(3): 346–50.

Cappelli M, MacDonald NE, McGrath PJ. Assessment of readiness to transfer to adult care for adolescents with cystic fibrosis. *Child Health Care.* 1989; **18**(4): 218–24.

Cavanaugh K, Wallston KA, Gebretsadik T, *et al.* Addressing literacy and numeracy to improve diabetes care: two randomized controlled trials. *Diabetes Care.* 2009; **32**(12): 2149–55.

Clarizia NA, Chahal N, Manlhiot C, *et al.* Transition to adult health care for adolescents and young adults with congenital heart disease: perspectives of the patient, parent and health care provider. *Can J Cardiol.* 2009; **25**(9): e317–22.

Crosnier H, Tubiana-Rufi N. [Modalities of transition of diabetic adolescents from pediatrics to the adult care in the Paris-Ile-de-France region: an appeal to cooperative work for improving quality of care. Paris-Ile-de-France Section of DESG (Diabetes Education Study Group) [French]. *Arch Pediatr.* 1998; **5**(12): 1327–33.

Cuttell K, Hilton D, Drew J. Preparation for transition to adult diabetes services. *Paediatr Nurs.* 2005; **17**(2): 28–30.

Dashiff C, Hardeman T, McLain R. Parent-adolescent communication and diabetes: an integrative review. *J Adv Nurs.* 2008a; **62**(2): 140–62.

Dashiff C, Vance D, Abdullatif H, *et al.* Parenting, autonomy and self-care of adolescents with type 1 diabetes. *Child Care Health Dev.* 2008b; **35**: 79–88.

Department of Health (DoH). *You're Welcome Quality Criteria: making health services young people friendly.* DoH; 2007.

Department of Health (DoH). *National Service Framework for Diabetes: standards.* DoH; 2001.

Department of Health (DoH) Diabetes Team. *Improving Diabetes Services: the NSF two years on; report from Dr Sue Roberts, National Clinical Director for Diabetes, to Secretary of State.* DoH; 2005.

Department of Health (DoH) Child Health and Maternity Services Branch. *Transition: getting it right for young people; improving the transition of young people with long term conditions from children's to adult health services.* Department for Education and Skills/DoH; 2006.

Dieppe CR, Kumar M, Crome I. Adolescent exploratory behavior: what do trainees know? *J Adolesc Health.* 2008; **43**(5): 520–2.

Donkervoort M, Wiegerink DJ, van Meeteren J, *et al.* Transition to adulthood: validation of the Rotterdam Transition Profile for young adults with cerebral palsy and normal intelligence. *Dev Med Child Neurol.* 2009; **51**(1): 53–62.

Dovey-Pearce G, Hurrell R, May C, *et al.* Young adults' (16–25 years) suggestions for providing developmentally appropriate diabetes services: a qualitative study. *Health Soc Care Community.* 2005; **13**(5): 409–19.

Dugueperoux I, Tamalet A, Sermet-Gaudelus I, *et al.* Clinical changes of patients with cystic fibrosis during transition from pediatric to adult care. *J Adolesc Health.* 2008; **43**(5): 459–65.

Durst CL, Horn MV, MacLaughlin EF, *et al.* Psychosocial responses of adolescent cystic fibrosis patients to lung transplantation. *Pediatr Transplant.* 2001; **5**(1): 27–31.

Eiser C, Flynn M, Green E, *et al.* Coming of age with diabetes: patients' views of a clinic for under-25 year olds. *Diabet Med.* 1993; **10**(3): 285–9.

Forbes A, While A, Ullman R, *et al.* Multimethod review to identify components of practice which may promote continuity in the transition from child to adult care for young people with chronic illness or disability. London: National Coordinating Centre for NHS Service Delivery and Organisation; 2001.

Frank M. Factors associated with non-compliance with a medical follow-up regimen after discharge from a pediatric diabetes clinic. *Can J Diabetes Care.* 1996; **20**: 14–20.

Fredericks EM, Dore-Stites D, Well A, *et al.* Assessment of transition readiness skills and adherence in pediatric liver transplant recipients. *Pediatr Transplant.* 2010; **14**(8): 944–53.

Frey MA, Guthrie B, Loveland-Cherry C, *et al.* Risky behavior and risk in adolescents with IDDM. *J Adolesc Health.* 1997; **20**(1): 38–45.

Geenen SJ, Powers LE, Sells W. Understanding the role of health care providers during the transition of adolescents with disabilities and special health care needs. *J Adolesc Health.* 2003; **32**(3): 225–33.

Geerts E, van de Wiel H, Tamminga R. A pilot study on the effects of the transition of paediatric to adult health care in patients with haemophilia and in their parents: patient and parent worries, parental illness-related distress and health-related quality of life. *Haemophilia.* 2008; **14**(5): 1007–13.

Goldenring J, Rosen D. Getting into adolescent heads: an essential update. *Contemp Pediatr.* 2004; **21**: 64–90.

Gosden C, Edge JA, Holt RI, *et al.* The fifth UK paediatric diabetes services survey: meeting guidelines and recommendations. *Arch Dis Child.* 2010; **95**(10): 837–40.

Griffin SJ. Lost to follow-up: the problem of defaulters from diabetes clinics. *Diabet Med.* 1998; **15**(Suppl. 3): S14–24.

Hambly H, Robling M, Crowne E, *et al.* Communication skills of healthcare professionals in paediatric diabetes services. *Diabet Med.* 2009; **26**(5): 502–9.

Hilderson D, Saidi AS, Van Deyk K, *et al.* Attitude toward and current practice of transfer and transition of adolescents with congenital heart disease in the United States of America and Europe. *Pediatr Cardiol.* 2009; **30**(6): 786–93.

Holmes-Walker DJ, Llewellyn AC, Farrell K. A transition care programme which improves diabetes control and reduces hospital admission rates in young adults with Type 1 diabetes aged 15–25 years. *Diabet Med.* 2007; **24**(7): 764–9.

International Society for Paediatric and Adolescent Diabetes (ISPAD). *Consensus Guidelines for the Management of Type 1 Diabetes in Children and Adolescents.* ISPAD; 2000.

Ivey JB, Wright A, Dashiff CJ. Finding the balance: adolescents with type 1 diabetes and their parents. *J Pediatr Health Care.* 2009; **23**(1): 10–18.

Johnson SB, Blum RW, Giedd JN. Adolescent maturity and the brain: the promise and pitfalls of neuroscience research in adolescent health policy. *J Adolesc Health.* 2009; 45(3): 216–21.

Jones K, Hammerlsey S, Shepherd M. Meeting the needs of young people with diabetes: an ongoing challenge. *J Diabetes Nurs.* 2003; 7: 345–50.

Kennedy A, Sawyer S. Transition from pediatric to adult services: are we getting it right? *Curr Opin Pediatr.* 2008; 20(4): 403–9.

Kennedy I. *Getting It Right for Children and Young People: overcoming cultural barriers in the NHS so as to meet their needs.* National Health Service; 2010.

Key JD, Marsh LD, Darden PM. Adolescent medicine in pediatric practice: a survey of practice and training. *Am J Med Sci.* 1995; 309(2): 83–7.

Kieckhefer GM, Trahms CM. Supporting development of children with chronic conditions: from compliance toward shared management. *Pediatr Nurs.* 2000; 26(4): 354–63.

Kipps S, Bahu T, Ong K, *et al.* Current methods of transfer of young people with Type 1 diabetes to adult services. *Diabet Med.* 2002; 19(8): 649–54.

Klostermann BK, Slap GB, Nebrig DM, *et al.* Earning trust and losing it: adolescents' views on trusting physicians. *J Fam Pract.* 2005; 54(8): 679–87.

Lam PY, Fitzgerald BB, Sawyer SM. Young adults in children's hospitals: why are they there? *Med J Aust.* 2005; 182(8): 381–4.

Lotstein DS, Ghandour R, Cash A, *et al.* Planning for health care transitions: results from the 2005–2006 National Survey of Children with Special Health Care Needs. *Pediatrics.* 2009; 123(1): e145–52.

Lotstein DS, McPherson M, Strickland B, *et al.* Transition planning for youth with special health care needs: results from the National Survey of Children with Special Health Care Needs. *Pediatrics.* 2005; 115(6): 1562–8.

Lurie S, Shemesh E, Sheiner PA, *et al.* Non-adherence in pediatric liver transplant recipients: an assessment of risk factors and natural history. *Pediatr Transplant.* 2000; 4(3): 200–6.

Lustig JL, Ozer EM, Adams SH, *et al.* Improving the delivery of adolescent clinical preventive services through skills-based training. *Pediatrics.* 2001; 107(5): 1100–7.

Luyckx K, Seiffge-Krenke I, Schwartz SJ, *et al.* Identity development, coping, and adjustment in emerging adults with a chronic illness: the sample case of type 1 diabetes. *J Adolesc Health.* 2008; 43(5): 451–8.

Middleman AB, Binns HJ, Durant RH. Factors affecting pediatric residents' intentions to screen for high risk behaviors. *J Adolesc Health.* 1995; 17(2): 106–12.

McDonagh JE, Shaw KL, Southwood TR. Growing up and moving on in rheumatology: development and preliminary evaluation of a transitional care programme for a multicentre cohort of adolescents with juvenile idiopathic arthritis. *J Child Health Care.* 2006; 10(1): 22–42.

McDonagh JE, Southwood TR, Shaw KL. The impact of a coordinated transitional care programme on adolescents with juvenile idiopathic arthritis. *Rheumatology (Oxford).* 2007; 46(1): 161–8.

McLaughlin SE, Diener-West M, Indurkhya A, *et al.* Improving transition from pediatric to adult cystic fibrosis care: lessons from a national survey of current practices. *Pediatrics.* 2008; 121(5): e1160–6.

McPherson M, Thaniel L, Minniti CP. Transition of patients with sickle cell disease from pediatric to adult care: Assessing patient readiness. *Pediatr Blood Cancer.* 2009; 52(7): 838–41.

Mellinger DC. Preparing students with diabetes for life at college. *Diabetes Care.* 2003; **26**(9): 2675–8.

Moons P, Pinxten S, Dedroog D, *et al.* Expectations and experiences of adolescents with congenital heart disease on being transferred from pediatric cardiology to an adult congenital heart disease program. *J Adolesc Health.* 2009; **44**(4): 316–22.

Mulvaney SA, Rothman RL, Osborn CY, *et al.* Self-management problem solving for adolescents with type 1 diabetes: intervention processes associated with an Internet program. *Patient Educ Couns.* Epub 2010a Oct 27.

Mulvaney SA, Rothman RL, Wallston KA, *et al.* An internet-based program to improve self-management in adolescents with type 1 diabetes. *Diabetes Care.* 2010b; **33**(3): 602–4.

Murphey DA, Lamonda KH, Carney JK, *et al.* Relationships of a brief measure of youth assets to health-promoting and risk behaviors. *J Adolesc Health.* 2004; **34**(3): 184–91.

Nakhla M, Daneman D, Frank M, *et al.* Translating transition: a critical review of the diabetes literature. *J Pediatr Endocrinol Metab.* 2008; **21**(6): 507–16.

Nakhla M, Daneman D, To T, *et al.* Transition to adult care for youths with diabetes mellitus: findings from a Universal Health Care System. *Pediatrics.* 2009; **124**(6): e1134–41.

National Institute for Clinical Excellence, National Collaborating Centre for Women's and Children's Health, National Collaborating Centre for Chronic Conditions. *Type 1 Diabetes: diagnosis and management of type 1 diabetes in children, young people and adults.* London: NICE; 1994.

Olsson CA, Bond L, Burns JM, *et al.* Adolescent resilience: a concept analysis. *J Adolesc.* 2003; **26**(1): 1–11.

Orr DP, Fineberg NS, Gray DL. Glycemic control and transfer of health care among adolescents with insulin dependent diabetes mellitus. *J Adolesc Health.* 1996; **18**(1): 44–7.

Pacaud D, McConnell B, Huot C. Transition from pediatric care to adult care for insulin-dependent diabetes patients. *Can J Diabetes Care.* 1996; **20**: 14–20.

Pacaud D, Yale JF, Stephure D, *et al.* Problems in transition from pediatric care to adult care for individuals with diabetes. *Can J Diabetes Care.* 2005; **29**: 13–18.

Perry L, Steinbeck KS, Dunbabin JS, *et al.* Lost in transition? Access to and uptake of adult health services and outcomes for young people with type 1 diabetes in regional New South Wales. *Med J Aust.* 2010; **193**(8): 444–9.

Reid GJ, Irvine MJ, McCrindle BW, *et al.* Prevalence and correlates of successful transfer from pediatric to adult health care among a cohort of young adults with complex congenital heart defects. *Pediatrics.* 2004; **113**(3 Pt. 1): e197–205.

Robertson LP, McDonagh JE, Southwood TR, *et al.* Growing up and moving on: a multicentre UK audit of the transfer of adolescents with juvenile idiopathic arthritis from paediatric to adult centred care. *Ann Rheum Dis.* 2006; **65**(1): 74–80.

Salmi J, Huupponen T, Oksa H, *et al.* Metabolic control in adolescent insulin-dependent diabetics referred from pediatric to adult clinic. *Ann Clin Res.* 1986; **18**(2): 84–7.

Sanci L, Coffey C, Patton G, *et al.* Sustainability of change with quality general practitioner education in adolescent health: a 5-year follow-up. *Med Educ.* 2005; **39**(6): 557–60.

Sanci LA, Coffey CM, Veit FC, *et al.* Evaluation of the effectiveness of an educational intervention for general practitioners in adolescent health care: randomised controlled trial. *BMJ.* 2000; **320**(7229): 224–30.

Sawicki GS, Lukens-Bull K, Yin X, *et al.* Measuring the transition readiness of youth with special healthcare needs: Validation of the TRAQ; Transition Readiness Assessment Questionnaire. *J Pediatr Psychol.* 2011; **36**(2): 160–71.

Scal P, Horvath K, Garwick A. Preparing for adulthood: health care transition counseling for youth with arthritis. *Arthritis Rheum.* 2009; **61**(1): 52–7.

Schilling LS, Knafl KA, Grey M. Changing patterns of self-management in youth with type I diabetes. *J Pediatr Nurs.* 2006; **21**(6): 412–24.

Shaw KL, Southwood TR, McDonagh JE. Young people's satisfaction of transitional care in adolescent rheumatology in the UK. *Child Care Health Dev.* 2007; **33**(4): 368–79.

Singh SP, Paul M, Ford T, *et al.* Transitions of care from Child and Adolescent Mental Health Services to Adult Mental Health Services (TRACK Study): a study of protocols in Greater London. *BMC Health Serv Res.* 2008; **8**: 135.

Stabile L, Rosser L, Porterfield KM, *et al.* Transfer versus transition: success in pediatric transplantation brings the welcome challenge of transition. *Prog Transplant.* 2005; **15**(4): 363–70.

Steinberg L. A behavioral scientist looks at the science of adolescent brain development. *Brain Cogn.* 2010; **72**(1): 160–4.

Steinkamp G, Ullrich G, Muller C, *et al.* Transition of adult patients with cystic fibrosis from paediatric to adult care: the patients' perspective before and after start-up of an adult clinic. *Eur J Med Res.* 2001; **6**(2): 85–92.

Stilley CS, Lawrence K, Bender A, *et al.* Maturity and adherence in adolescent and young adult heart recipients. *Pediatr Transplant.* 2006; **10**(3): 323–30.

Surís JC, Akre C, Rutishauser C. How adult specialists deal with the principles of a successful transition. *J Adolesc Health.* 2009; **45**(6): 551–5.

Surís JC, Michaud PA, Akre C, *et al.* Health risk behaviors in adolescents with chronic conditions. *Pediatrics.* 2008; **122**(5): e1113–18.

Tuchman LK, Slap GB, Britto MT. Transition to adult care: experiences and expectations of adolescents with a chronic illness. *Child Care Health Dev.* 2008; **34**(5): 557–63.

Van Staa A, van der Stege HA, Jedeloo S, *et al.* Readiness to transfer to adult care of adolescents with chronic conditions: exploration of associated factors. *J Adolesc Health.* 2011; **48**(3): 295–302.

Van Walleghem N, Macdonald CA, Dean HJ. Evaluation of a systems navigator model for transition from pediatric to adult care for young adults with type 1 diabetes. *Diabetes Care.* 2008; **31**(8): 1529–30.

Vanelli M, Caronna S, Adinolfi B, *et al.* Effectiveness of an uninterrupted procedure to transfer adolescents with type 1 diabetes from the Paediatric to the Adult Clinic held in the same hospital: eight-year experience with the Parma protocol. *Diabetes Nutr Metab.* 2004; **17**(5): 304–8.

Watanabe A, Shaw KL, Rankin E, *et al.* Young people's expectations of and satisfaction with transitional care from paediatric and adult care perspectives. *Arch Dis Child.* 2010; **95**(Suppl. 1): A65.

Weissberg-Benchell J, Wolpert H, Anderson BJ. Transitioning from pediatric to adult care: a new approach to the post-adolescent young person with type 1 diabetes. *Diabetes Care.* 2007; **30**(10): 2441–6.

While A, Forbes A, Ullman R, *et al.* Good practices that address continuity during transition from child to adult care: synthesis of the evidence. *Child Care Health Dev.* 2004; **30**(5): 439–52.

Wiener LS, Zobel M, Battles H, *et al.* Transition from a pediatric HIV intramural clinical research program to adolescent and adult community-based care services: assessing transition readiness. *Soc Work Health Care.* 2007; **46**(1): 1–19.

Williams T, Sherman E, Mah J, *et al.* Measurement of medical self-management and transition readiness among Canadian adolescents with special health care needs. *Int J Child Adolesc Health*. 2010; **3**: 1–9.

Wolff K, Cavanaugh K, Malone R, *et al*. The Diabetes Literacy and Numeracy Education Toolkit (DLNET): materials to facilitate diabetes education and management in patients with low literacy and numeracy skills. *Diabetes Educ*. 2009; **35**(2): 233–6, 238–41, 244–5.

Wolfstadt J, Kaufman A, Levitin J, *et al*. The use and usefulness of MyHealth passport: an online tool for the creation of a portable health summary. *Int J Child Adolesc Health*. 2010; **3**(4): 499–506.

Woods E, Neinstein L. Office visit, interview techniques and recommendations. In: Neinstein L, Gordon C, Katzman D, *et al.*, editors. *Adolescent Health Care: a practical guide*. 5th ed. Philadelphia: Lippincott Williams & Wilkins; 2008. pp. 32–44.

Wysocki T, Hough BS, Ward KM, *et al*. Diabetes mellitus in the transition to adulthood: adjustment, self-care, and health status. *J Dev Behav Pediatr*. 1992; **13**(3): 194–201.

Yeo MS, Bond LM, Sawyer SM. Health risk screening in adolescents: room for improvement in a tertiary inpatient setting. *Med J Aust*. 2005; **183**(8): 427–9.

Zack J, Jacobs CP, Keenan PM, *et al*. Perspectives of patients with cystic fibrosis on preventive counseling and transition to adult care. *Pediatr Pulmonol*. 2003; **36**(5): 376–83.

PART III

Tools for Clinical Practice

Diagnostic tools for children

Susie Colville

The following is a comprehensive but not exhaustive list of clinical tools that can be used to assess behaviour, depression, anxiety and quality of life in young people. Clinical assessment by experienced clinical staff can be accompanied by referral to a clinical psychologist or psychiatrist for a more formal assessment.

GENERAL BEHAVIOUR

The *Child Behaviour Checklist (CBCL)* (Achenbach, 1991, 1992) can be used to measure internalising (e.g. anxious, depressive) behaviours and externalising (e.g. aggressive, hyperactive) behaviours that may be associated with a range of emotional and behavioural difficulties, in children and young people aged between 1½ and 18 years. The CBCL is made up of two sections: the first section contains 20 items assessing competence; the second section consists of 120 items to assess emotional and behavioural difficulties in the past 6 months. Parents, caregivers, teachers and young people can fill out the checklist.

The *Strengths and Difficulties Questionnaire (SDQ)* (Goodman, 1997) is a behavioural screening questionnaire for children aged between 3 and 16 years. There are parent and teacher versions and also a youth self-report version for young people aged 11 years and over. The SDQ is made up of 25 items divided among five scales: (i) emotional difficulties; (ii) behavioural difficulties; (iii) hyperactivity; (iv) peer relationship difficulties; and (v) pro-social behaviours. More recent versions (Goodman, 1999) also contain an impact supplement that can be used to assess the impact of identified difficulties on the young person's life. SDQ can help identify risks of developing an emotional, behavioural or inattention disorder in young people.

MEASURES FOR DEPRESSION

The National Institute for Health and Clinical Excellence (NICE, 2005) guidelines recommend a stepped-care model for depression in children and adolescents. The stepped-care approach involves 'a sequence of treatment options offering simpler and less expensive interventions first and more complex and expensive interventions if the patient has not benefited, based on locally agreed protocols' (NICE 2005, CG28, page 67). Questionnaire measures designed to assess depressive symptoms in young people could therefore be used as part of the initial stages of a stepped-care approach.

The *Mood and Feelings Questionnaire (MFQ)* (Angold and Costello, 1987; Angold *et al.* 1995) is made up of a series of 34 short statement items (13 in the short version) designed to assess how young people aged between 13 and 18 years have been feeling or acting recently, in order to detect clinical depression in this population. The MFQ also includes parent and teacher forms made up of 33 items (13 in the short version).

The *Multiscore Depression Inventory for Adolescents and Adults (MDI)* is a self-report tool made up of 118 true/false statements designed to identify indicators of depression in young people aged 13 years and over. (Berndt 1986) A shorter version of the MDI, made up of 49 items, is also available.

The *Multiscore Depression Inventory for Children (MDI-C)* is for use with children aged between 8 and 12 years and is made up of 79 true/false statements (Berndt and Petzel, 1980).

The *Child Depression Inventory (CDI)* is a 27-item self-report tool designed to measure cognitive, affective and behavioural indicators of depression in young people between the ages of 7 and 17 years (Carey *et al.*, 1987).

The *Reynolds Child Depression Scale (RCDS)* for ages 8–12 and the *Reynolds Adolescent Depression Scale (2nd ed, RADS-2)* for ages 11–20 (Reynolds 1989, 2002). Each self-report scale is made up of 30 items designed to screen for different categories of depressive symptoms.

Beck Depression Inventory for Youth (BDI-Y) is a 20-item self-report to detect early symptoms of depression in children aged between 7 and 14 years (Beck *et al.* 2001). The *Beck Depression Inventory (BDI-II)* has 21 items and can be used with adolescents aged 13 years and over (Beck 1961, Beck *et al.* 1996).

The *Children's Depression Scale (CDS)* was designed to assess depressed feelings and behaviour in young people aged between 7 and 18 years. The measure consists of 10 items. Parent/teacher versions are made up of 50 items (Lang and Tisher, 1978, 1987).

The *Center for Epidemiological Studies Depression Scale for Children (CES-DC)* is a 20-item self-report rating scale to measure current level of depressive symptoms and can be completed by children between the ages of 6 and 17 years (Weissman *et al.*, 1980).

The *WHO-5 Well-Being Index* is a short questionnaire containing five positively worded statements designed to capture a young person's emotional well-being over the previous 2 weeks (*see* Table A). It offers the possibility to screen for mood changes at regular intervals and in general practice. This web-based questionnaire may offer new and faster opportunities to identify pathological changes in emotional well-being and may lead to earlier therapeutic interventions (www.who-5.org; Bech, 2004).

TABLE A: WHO–5: A VALIDATED TOOL TO SCREEN WELL-BEING

Please indicate for each of the five statements which is closest to how you have been feeling over the last 2 weeks.

	All of the time	Most of the time	More than half of the time	Less than half of the time	Some of the time	At no time
I have felt cheerful and in good spirits						
I have felt calm and relaxed						
I have felt active and vigorous						
I have woken up feeling fresh and rested						
My daily life has been filled with things that interest me						

MEASURES FOR ANXIETY

A well-used measure of anxiety is the *State Trait Anxiety Inventory for Children (STAIC)*. This self-report tool made up of 20 items is designed to assess temperament-based (trait) anxiety and current-level (state) anxiety in children aged between 8 and 14 years (Spielberger 1973).

The *Spence Children's Anxiety Scale (SCAS)* consists of 44 items designed to assess anxiety symptoms in children aged 8–12 years (Spence 1998).

The *Multidimensional Anxiety Scale for Children (MASC)* contains 39 items designed to measure different areas of anxiety in young people aged between 8 and 19 years. The short-scale version *(MASC-10)* consists of only 10 items and is designed for repeat testing in order to track a young person's progress (March 1997).

The *Beck Anxiety Inventory for Youth (BAI-Y)* is a 20-item self-report measure that can be used with children and adolescents between the ages of 7 and 14 years to identify specific fears and worries, as well as physiological symptoms associated with anxiety (Beck *et al.* 2001).

These general measures will not be able to identify specific worries around diabetes complications or care, which is why specific diabetes-related questionnaires have been developed as well.

Diabetes-specific anxiety measures

The *Hypoglycemia Fear Survey (HFS)* was developed for use in adults with diabetes by Cox *et al.* (1987). Green *et al.* (1990) evaluated the psychometric properties of this measure in a diabetic youth population. The HFS is made up of 23 items and can be used to assess fear relating to hypoglycaemia in children/adolescents with type 1 diabetes mellitus and their parents. There are two subscales: a worry subscale and a behaviour subscale.

The *Hypoglycemia Fear Survey parent scale (HFS-P)* is made up of 25 items and can be used with parents of preadolescent/adolescents with type 1 diabetes mellitus (Clarke *et al.* 1998).

The *Hypoglycemia Fear Survey parent of young children scale (HFS-P-YC)* is made up of 26 items and is for use with parents of younger children with type 1 diabetes mellitus (Patton *et al.*, 2008).

Barnard *et al.* (2010) suggest that fear of hypoglycaemia can be significantly under-reported. Therefore, the HFS could be used to identify when additional support from the diabetes team may be appropriate.

It is also important to address anxiety in parents and to consider how this anxiety expresses itself in the family.

The *Paediatric Inventory for Parents (PIP)* was developed by the Children's Hospital of Philadelphia (Streisand *et al.*, 2000) and was originally evaluated within a paediatric oncology setting. The tool is a 42-item self-report measure designed to assess illness-related parenting stress in parents of children and adolescents having been treated or having ongoing treatment for a chronic illness. There are four domains: (i) 'communication' (e.g. arguments with family members, speaking with doctors/child about illness); (ii) 'emotional functioning' (e.g. learning upsetting news); (iii) 'medical care' (e.g. making decisions about medical treatment); and (iv) 'role function' (e.g. being unable to go to work, attending to needs of family members).

Several measures of quality of life include questions about worries and general anxiety.

MEASURES FOR QUALITY OF LIFE

KIDSCREEN-10 (Ravens-Sieberer *et al.*, 2005) is a 27-item self-report measure of health-related quality of life that can be completed by children and adolescents aged between 8 and 18 years and it takes only 5 minutes to complete. There are also two longer measures (*KIDSCREEN-27* and *KIDSCREEN-52*), which can be used to develop a more detailed profile of health-related quality of life across a maximum of 10 dimensions.

The *Pediatric Quality of Life Inventory/Questionnaire (PedsQL)* (Varni *et al.*, 1999) is made up of 15 core items. It is a generic tool to measure health-related quality of life in children, but it also includes a diabetes-specific module. Designed for children aged between 2 and 18 years (children aged under 5 are assessed via a proxy report from the parent/carer).

The *Diabetes Quality of Life questionnaire for Youths (DQOL-Y)* (Ingersoll and Marrero, 1991) is made up of three subscales, each designed to assess the impact of diabetes on different areas of a young person's life: (i) diabetes life satisfaction (17 items); (ii) impact of diabetes (23 items); and (iii) diabetes-related worries (11 items). The questionnaire is for use with adolescents aged between 11 and 18 years. The DQOL was used in the Diabetes Control and Complications Trial. The Hvidoere Study Group used the youth version. These measures are designed to measure specific diabetes-related challenges (Skinner *et al.*, 2006).

The *Revised children's quality of life questionnaire (KINDL-R)* (Ravens-Sieberer and Bullinger, 1998) involves 24 items designed to assess health-related quality of life in children. There are three different age groups (4–7, 8–11 and 12–16 years) and also parent versions of each. The KINDL-R contains disease-specific modules, including one for diabetes.

The *Netherlands Organisation for Applied Scientific Research Child Quality of Life Questionnaire (TACQOL)* (Vogels *et al.*, 1998; Verrips *et al.*, 1998) is a 56-item inventory. It offers young people the opportunity to differentiate between their physical functioning and how they feel about it. It is designed for use with children aged from 8 to 15 years with chronic medical conditions. There is also a parent form – parents can act as a proxy for children aged 6 years and over.

EU-DISABKIDS (Bullinger *et al.*, 2002; Baars *et al.*, 2005) is a recently developed European project with the aim of 'improving quality of life and independence in young people with chronic medical conditions'.[1] A number of questionnaires (core instruments and disease-specific modules) have been developed as part of the project in order to assess health-related quality of life in young people aged 4–16 years across Europe. There are seven separate disease modules for common chronic medical conditions, of which one is diabetes. The diabetes module is made up of two separate scales: impact and treatment. 'The Impact scale describes emotional reactions of needing to control every day life, and to restrict one's diet, the Treatment scale refers to carrying equipment and planning treatment'.[2]

The *Well-Being Questionnaire (W-BQ 12 (short form), W-BQ 22 and W-BQ 28 (diabetes specific))* (Speight *et al.*, 2000) is for use to assess psychological well-being in adults and adolescents with diabetes aged 16 years and over. The *W-BQ 28* is a diabetes-specific measure. (*W-BQ 12*: subscales – positive well-being, energy and negative well-being; *W-BQ 22*: subscales – depression, anxiety, energy and positive well-being; *W-BQ 28*: subscales – generic negative well-being, energy, generic positive well-being, generic stress, diabetes-specific negative well-being, diabetes-specific stress, diabetes-specific positive well-being.)

It is important to remember that these measures are not 'diagnostic'; rather, they are screening tools to help healthcare professionals, families and young people think about whether additional assessment and support is needed (Canning and Kelleher, 1994). Clinical experience and observation by the diabetes team may indicate where further evaluation would be helpful.

It is also important to note that responses may be affected by the way these measures are administered. The wish to please the interviewer can create differences in self-reported and interview-based questionnaires, which could lead to an underestimation of emotional or behavioural difficulties (Horsch *et al.*, 2007).

DIABETES-RELATED DISTRESS (NOT CHILD-SPECIFIC)

The *Problem Areas In Diabetes (PAID)* scale (Polonsky *et al.*, 1995) is a widely used measure of the range of emotional responses to diabetes. It is composed of 20 items designed to assess a range of problems commonly reported in type 1 and type 2 diabetes.

The *Diabetes Distress Scale (DDS)* (Polonsky *et al.*, 2005) is a 17-item measure designed to assess diabetes-related emotional distress across four domains: (i) emotional burden; (ii) physician-related distress; (iii) regimen-related

---

1 EU-DISABKIDS website: www.disabkids.de/cms/thedisabkidsproject
2 EU-DISABKIDS Information on the Diabetes Module: www.disabkids.de/cms/module_diabetes

distress; and (iv) diabetes-related interpersonal distress. A brief two-item version of the DDS has since been developed (Fisher *et al.*, 2008) to act as a screener for the 17-item DDS, for use in clinical settings.

The *Questionnaire on Stress in patients with Diabetes Revised (QSD-R)* (Herschbach *et al.*, 1997) is a diabetes-specific tool and is a shortened version of the original QSD (Duran *et al.*, 1995). It is made up of 45 items designed to identify areas of stress using eight different stress scales: (i) leisure time; (ii) depression/fear of future; (iii) hypoglycaemia; (iv) treatment regimen/diet; (v) physical complaints; (vi) work; (vii) partner; and (viii) doctor–patient relationship.

TREATMENT SATISFACTION

The *Diabetes Treatment Satisfaction Questionnaire (status version, DTSQs)* (Bradley, 1994) is made up of eight items that provide the capacity to assess overall diabetes treatment satisfaction, treatment satisfaction in specific areas, and perceived frequencies of hyperglycaemia and hypoglycaemia in young people living with diabetes, and their parents.

REFERENCES

Achenbach T. *Manual for the Child Behavior Checklist/4–18 and 1991 Profile*. Burlington, VT: University of Vermont Department of Psychiatry; 1991.

Achenbach T. *Manual for the Child Behavior Checklist/2–3 and 1992 Profile*. Burlington, VT: University of Vermont Department of Psychiatry; 1992.

Angold A, Costello EJ. *Mood and feelings questionnaire (MFQ)*. Durham: Duke University, Developmental Epidemiology Program; 1987.

Angold A., Costello EJ, Messer SC. *et al.* Development of a short questionnaire for use in epidemiological studies of depression in children and adolescents. *Int J Methods Psychiatr Res.* 1995; 5: 237–49.

Baars RM, Atherton CI, Koopman HM, *et al.* The European DISABKIDS project: development of seven condition-specific modules to measure health related quality of life in children and adolescents. *Health Qual Life Outcomes.* 2005; 3: 70.

Barnard K, Thomas S, Royle P, *et al.* Fear of hypoglycaemia in parents of young children with type 1 diabetes: a systematic review. *BMC Pediatr.* 2010; **10**: 50–60.

Bech P. Measuring the dimensions of psychological general well-being by the WHO-5. *QoL Newsletter.* 2004; **32**: 15–16.

Beck JS, Beck AT, Jolly JB. *Beck Youth Inventories*. San Antonio, TX, USA: The Psychological Corporation. 2001.

Beck AT. *Beck Depression Inventory*. Philadelphia, PA, USA: Center for Cognitive Therapy, 1961.

Beck AT, Steer RA, Brown GK. *Manual for the Beck Depression Inventory-II*. San Antonio, TX: Psychological Corporation; 1996.

Berndt DJ. *Multiscore Depression Inventory (MDI) Manual*. Los Angeles: Western Psychological Services; 1986.

Berndt DJ, Petzel TP. Development and initial evaluation of a multiscore depression inventory. *J Pers Assess.* 1980; **44**(4): 396–403.

Bradley C. *Diabetes treatment satisfaction questionnaire. Handbook of Psychology and Diabetes.* Chur, Switzerland: Harwood Academic Publishers; 1994; 111–32.

Bullinger M, Schmidt S, Petersen C, *et al.* Assessing quality of life of children with chronic health conditions and disabilities: a European approach. *Int J Rehabil Res.* 2002; **25**(3): 197–206.

Canning, E, Kelleher K. Performance of screening tools for mental health problems in chronically ill children. *Arch Pediatr Adolesc Med.* 1994; **148**(3): 272–8.

Carey MP, Haulstich ME, Gresham FM, *et al.* Children's Depression Inventory construct and discriminant validity across clinical and non referred (control) populations. *J Consul Clin Psychol.* 1987; **55**: 755–61.

Clarke WL, Gonder-Frederick A, Snyder AL, *et al.* Maternal fear of hypoglycemia in their children with insulin dependent diabetes mellitus. *J Pediatr Endocrinol Metab.* 1998; **11**(1): 189–94.

Cox DJ, Irvine A, Gonder-Frederick L, *et al.* Fear of hypoglycaemia: quantification, validation and utilization. *Diabetes Care.* 1987; **10**(5): 617–21.

Duran G, Herschbach P, Waadt S, *et al.* Assessing daily problems with diabetes: a subject-oriented approach to compliance. *Psychol Rep.* 1995; **76**(2): 515–21.

EU-DISABKIDS. www.disabkids.de/cms/thedisabkidsproject

EU-DISABKIDS Information on the Diabetes Module: www.disabkids.de/cms/module_diabetes

Fisher L, Glasgow RE, Mullan JT, *et al.* 2008. Development of a brief diabetes distress screening instrument. *Ann Fam Med.* 2008; **6**(3): 246–52.

Green LB, Wysocki T, Reineck BM. Fear of hypoglycemia in children and adolescents with diabetes. *J Pediatr Psychol.* 1990; **15**: 633–41.

Goodman R. The Strengths and Difficulties Questionnaire: a research note. *J Child Psychol Psychiatry.* 1997; **38**(5): 581–6.

Goodman R. The extended version of the Strengths and Difficulties Questionnaire as a guide to child psychiatric caseness and consequent burden. *J Child Psychol Psychiatry.* 1999; **40**(5): 791–801.

Herschbach P, Duran G, Waadt S, *et al.* Psychometric properties of the Questionnaire on Stress in Patients with Diabetes – Revised (QSD-R). *Health Psychol.* 1997; **16**(2): 171–4.

Horsch A, McManus F, Kennedy P, *et al.* Anxiety, depressive, and posttraumatic stress symptoms in mothers of children with type 1 diabetes. *J Trauma Stress.* 2007; **20**(5): 881–91.

Ingersoll GM, Marrero DG. A modified quality-of-life measure for youths: psychometric properties. *Diabetes Educ.* 1991; **17**(2): 114–18.

Lang M, Tisher M. *Childrens Depression Scale: research edition.* Melbourne: The Australian Council for Educational Research Limited; 1978.

Lang M, Tisher M. *Childrens Depression Scale Manual, North American edition.* Palo Alto, CA: Consulting Psychologists Press; 1987.

March JS. *Manual for the Multidimensional Anxiety Scale for Children (MASC).* New York, NY: Multi-Health Systems; 1997.

March JS. *Multidimensional Anxiety Scale for Children Short Version (MASC-10).* New York, NY: Multi-Health Systems; 1997.

National Institute for Health and Clinical Excellence (NICE) Clinical Guideline 28. *Depression in Children and Young People. Identification and Management in Primary, Community and Secondary Care.* Sept 2005.

NICE definition of 'Stepped-care model' CG28, page 67. Sept 2005.

Patton SR, Dolan LM, Henry R, *et al.* Fear of hypoglycemia in parents of young children with type 1 diabetes mellitus. *J Clin Psychol Med Settings.* 2008; **15**(3): 251–9.

Polonsky WH, Anderson BJ, Lohrer PA, *et al.* Assessment of diabetes-related distress. *Diabetes Care.* 1995; **18**(6): 754–60.

Polonsky WH, Fisher L, Earles J, *et al.* Assessing psychosocial stress in diabetes. *Diabetes Care.* 2005; **28**(3): 626–31.

Ravens-Sieberer U, Gosch A, Rajmil L, *et al.* KIDSCREEN-52 quality-of-life measure for children and adolescents. *Expert Rev Pharmacoecon Outcomes Res.* 2005; **5**(3): 353–64.

Ravens-Sieberer U, Bullinger M. Assessing health-related quality of life in chronically ill children with the German KINDL: first psychometric and content analytical results. *Qual Life Res.* 1998; **7**(5): 399–407.

Reynolds, WM. *Reynolds Child Depression Scale.* Odessa, FL: Psychological Assessment Resources; 1989.

Reynolds WM. *Reynolds Adolescent Depression Scale – 2nd Edition (RADS-2): professional manual.* Lutz, FL: PAR Psychological Assessment Resources; 2002.

Skinner TC, Hoey H, McGee HM *et al.* For the Hvidøre Study Group on Childhood Diabetes Diabetes Quality of Life for Youth – Short Form (DQOLY-SF). Exploratory and confirmatory analysis in a sample of 2077 young people with type 1 diabetes mellitus. *Diabetologia.* 2006; **49**(4): 621–3.

Spence SH. A measure of anxiety symptoms among children. *Beh Res Ther.* 1998; **36**: 545–66.

Speight J, Barendse S, Bradley C. The W-BQ 28: further development of the Well-Being Questionnaire to include diabetes-specific as well as generic subscales and new stress subscales. *Proc Br Psychol Soc.* 2000; **8**(1): 21.F.

Spielberger CD. *Manual for the State-Trait Anxiety Inventory for Children.* Palo Alto, CA: Consulting Psychologists Press; 1973.

Streisand R, Braniecki S, Tercyak KP, *et al.* Childhood illness-related parenting stress: the Paediatric Inventory for Parents. *J Paediatr Psychol.* 2000; **26**(3): 155–62.

Varni JW, Seid M, Rode CA. The PedsQL: measurement model for the pediatric quality of life inventory. *Med Care.* 1999; **37**(2): 126–39.

Vernps GH, Vogels AGC, Verloove-Vanhorick SP *et al.* Health-related quality of life measure for children: the TACQOL. *J Appl Therapeut.* 1998; **4**: 357–60.

Vogels AGC Verrips GH, Fekkes M *et al.* Young children's health related quality of life: development of the TACQOL. *Qual Life Res.* 1998; **7**: 457–65.

Weissman MM, Orvaschel H, Padian N. Children's symptom and social functioning self-report scales: comparison of mothers' and children's reports. *J Nerv Ment Disord.* 1980; **168**(12): 736–40.

Assessment and intervention for diabetes-related cognitive difficulties

Angela Griffin

MEASURING OVERALL INTELLECTUAL ABILITY

The Wechsler Intelligence Scale for Children (WISC) is most commonly used to measure overall intellectual ability. This is a broad-ranging measure containing several subtests assessing ability in a number of cognitive areas. The current version of the WISC (WISC-IV) provides a full-scale IQ, verbal IQ and performance IQ and can identify areas of strength and/or challenges across the range of cognitive functioning. The Verbal IQ is derived from scores on subtests assessing verbal comprehension and working memory. Verbal comprehension is a measure of the child's ability to think, reason and problem-solve using language; working memory involves attention to spoken information and the ability to hold information 'online' in memory while processing it. Performance IQ is derived from scores on subtests assessing perceptual organisation skills and processing speed. Perceptual organisation requires attention to visual details, the ability to construct whole designs from their parts, to understand pattern and visual sequencing and to mentally rotate objects. Processing speed measures the speed with which the student can work through simple or routine information without making errors and also requires motor speed.

Performance on the WISC-IV intelligence test can be used to predict how well a child should be achieving in literacy and numeracy tasks. Where there is a significant discrepancy, it is important to identify the cause, as this will dictate the type of support that will be most helpful. For example, the root of the problem may lie in one of a number of potential specific areas, such as working memory, phonological processing, visual processing, auditory processing or processing speed.

In busy classroom situations, it is not unusual for children who are performing at an average level to be overlooked when it comes to assessment of learning needs or for consideration of support strategies. Longitudinal monitoring of progress may highlight a relative drop in achievement over time from the top of the class when they were younger (pre-diagnosis) to the middle of the class a few years later. This slower-than-expected development can indicate an underlying cognitive difficulty that is gradually impacting on learning. Comparing the child with themselves over time is important in order to pick up on this and can be explored by the diabetes team by asking parents for a historical perspective. Difficulties are often highlighted at times of change to the workload, to the pace of learning or when there are expectations of independent learning. The key time points are typically in the upper years of primary school, at transfer to secondary school and at the beginning of the General Certificate of Secondary Education (GCSE) programme.

SPEED OF PROCESSING

Learning often involves a combination of routine information processing such as reading, along with more complex information processing such as reasoning. Therefore, a slower speed of processing can leave less time and mental energy for the complex task of understanding new material. If a child's processing speed is slower than the speed of their peers', this can have a direct impact on how well the child can keep up with explanations, instructions and work in class.

Holmes *et al.* (1985) found that children with diabetes of early onset (at under 7 years of age) and long duration (more than 5 years) did more poorly on the performance subtests of the WISC, although still within the average range. As the lower scores were not linked to any one subtest, it is suggested that generally slower responding meant the children did not earn time bonuses. In terms of day-to-day functioning, this may mean that children with early-onset/long-duration diabetes are at a disadvantage on timed tests or on any tasks with a time limit.

In primary school, there may be more leeway for repetition, and sometimes there is support available from teaching assistants. However, where this is not the case or in the faster-moving environment of the secondary school classroom, there may be a greater impact. As workload increases, it can also mean that homework takes longer than it should. If children consistently feel overwhelmed by workload, teachers and parents should question the possibility of slowed processing speed. If teachers find that the child's test performance is not as good as they expected in comparison with how they contribute in class, or if the child typically does not manage to complete all the questions they can answer in an exam situation, there may be an issue with processing speed.

Difficulty with processing speed means the child does not get an equal opportunity to demonstrate their knowledge base. Time allowances can help in this situation. Individual cognitive assessment may not always be necessary, but if it is suspected that a child is taking longer than expected to work their way through tasks, particularly in the early years, it is possible to perform some time sampling of their work in the class environment.

Processing speed	
Potential issues	*Strategies and supports*
Homework taking longer	Consider reducing homework where possible
	Provide written handouts of lessons
Not taking down notes quickly enough in class, e.g. homework	Ensure enough time to note homework tasks
Not showing all knowledge in timed situations, e.g. exams	Use time sampling in class to establish how much extra time is needed to provide a fair chance
	If necessary, request extra time allowance for state exams
Frustration: tendency to take shortcuts or to write a minimum	Reward quality of work, not just quantity
	Encourage touch typing; some children do better at typing, but not all

ATTENTION

Attention and concentration are the building blocks for all learning. Any deficit in attention will have a significant impact and will become increasingly apparent if demands are high, e.g. if the child needs to divide attention between two things at once. In the classroom, this can happen many times a day. For example, listening to the teacher speak while also taking down notes or homework from the board will mean that one or the other is missed, usually the homework notes. If the child has to screen out conversation among other children in order to focus on what the teacher is saying (selective attention), this may also put pressure on an attention system that is already functioning at its maximum. Continuing to pay attention to something they do not find engaging and ignoring distractions in order to do so (sustained attention) can also be particularly difficult. A common complaint of parents and teachers is that the child can pay attention well if they are interested in something, usually citing a Nintendo DS, Facebook or computer games. This does not rule out an attention difficulty, as those circumstances are the most supportive and least demanding of attentional skills. Any interactive system, such as computers, is particularly effective at masking attention difficulties, as the instant feedback demands attention and rewards attention in a continuous loop.

Attention	
Potential issues	*Strategies and supports*
Dividing attention	Only have to pay attention to one thing at a time; limit need for dual tasking
	Use short instructions and prompts
Selective attention: avoiding distraction	Limit distractions
	Sit child at front, perhaps with a studious buddy
	One-to-one teaching or small-group work when possible
Sustaining attention	Break tasks down into manageable chunks
	Short periods of concentration, vary tasks and teaching style
	Integrate movement breaks, e.g. give books out
	Use their name often, praise while still paying attention, change task before attention runs out

MEMORY

Memory and learning difficulties have an effect on new learning, particularly in children with early-onset diabetes (e.g. Holmes *et al.*, 1985). In the early years, this may be noticeable in difficulty learning times tables and in reading or listening comprehension tasks. If new learning is not laid down, this can have a cumulative effect, with the gap widening over the years. In this way, a relatively minor memory deficit can have a significant impact. When teachers frequently feel that a child has not been listening, consideration should be given to whether this implicates attentional and/or memory impairment.

A number of longitudinal research studies outline the potentially adverse effects of diabetes on verbal memory (Fox *et al.* 2003; Kovacs *et al.*, 1994; Northam *et al.* 2001). In the school setting, this may be noticeable as a lack of progress or a slowing in the expected rate of progress in a child's general learning and vocabulary development. As the differences may not be large, teachers may note in end-of-term reports that the child has the ability to 'do better if they apply themselves more next term'. Continually slipping grades that don't recover should serve as a cause for concern. Children who state a clear preference for 'doing' subjects that are language-light, such as maths, science experiments and physical education, and who struggle with subjects with a heavy language component, such as English and history, may also be experiencing difficulty with verbal memory.

Effects on verbal memory may also be noticeable in how well a young person can manage their diabetes treatment. Managing a diabetes treatment regimen has significant memory demands. Some are relatively simple, repetitive tasks, such as blood glucose monitoring, and others require more complex memory skills, such as ongoing calorie calculation throughout the day. Remembering and calculating continual daily carbohydrate consumption is a complex task and appears to rely on quantitative working memory Soutor *et al.* (2004). In adults with years of practice, many of these skills become 'automated' and require little thought. For adolescents who are taking more responsibility for their treatment, there will be a significant demand on memory.

Memory	
Potential issues	*Strategies and supports*
Holding information in mind in the short term	Use calculators for maths
	Encourage showing working out in maths to help keep track
Learning and remembering new information	Reduce distractions
	Repeat instructions and check they have been understood
Following a film or a story	Small amounts of new information at a time
	Support error-free learning; prompt enough to ensure they find correct answer
Remembering homework tasks or messages for home	Use diaries, checklists, phone to prompt memory
Remembering previous discussions	Provide scaffold for memory by providing lesson plan
Poor generalisation of information from one setting to another	Discuss lessons afterwards
	Provide written back-up
	Repetition and rehearsal
	Make connections between new information and things they already know about
Route finding, e.g. around new school	Use visual prompts in the environment
Elements of new sequenced tasks	Use prompt cards for sequenced tasks

EXECUTIVE FUNCTIONING

Executive function refers to the higher-order cognitive skills involved in initiating and planning activities, self-monitoring progress and adjusting appropriately, starting, finishing and changing from one activity to another, inhibiting wrong responses and flexible thinking. These are skills that continue to develop for the longest period of time and are related to frontal lobe development, which continues into adulthood. As such, if there is a difficulty in the area of executive function, it will not always be fully apparent until the age at which these skills are expected to emerge, usually in the middle child-hood and teenage years. Executive functioning deficits may go unnoticed until this time, and even then they may be attributed to immaturity or children may be described as 'late developers'. The kinds of problems experienced in school can include not taking responsibility for coursework, missing deadlines, poor organisation, doing things impulsively or at the last minute, getting sidetracked and seeming to miss the point in an essay or in exam answers. These organis-ing, thinking ahead and planning skills are also important in the independent management of diabetes.

Direct investigation of school problems in individuals with type 1 diabetes mellitus are necessary to determine any relationship with the cognitive impair-ments described in the research. This practical information would also allow doctors and parents to give appropriate weight to these findings in making treatment decisions for children with type 1 diabetes mellitus.

Executive function	
Potential issues	Strategies and supports
Planning	Provide structure and prompts and gradually fade them out over time
	Use mind-mapping or similar to help with revision and with planning essays
Organising	Give structure or overview of lesson beforehand
	Practise use of timetables, wall calendars, whiteboards to assist with planning for short-term and longer-term deadlines
Self-monitoring	Work on using Filofax or mobile phone to provide reminders, prompts, etc.
	Model and reward checking of work
Initiating tasks or communication	One-to-one planning sessions to review and to troubleshoot
	Clear expectations and feedback
	Realistic goals
Problem-solving	Model step-by-step approach to problem-solving using their own real-life situations

PERCEPTUAL SKILLS

'There is some evidence that type 1 diabetes can have an effect on percep-tual skills, particularly where this a history of hyperglycaemia and ketonuria (Ferguson *et al.*, 2003, Rovet *et al.*, 1990). While these may be difficult to pick up on in the classroom, they may have a subtle but significant effect. It may be observed as untidy classwork or homework, disorganisation or disorientation.'

Perceptual skills

Potential issues	Strategies and supports
Spatial awareness: transferring 2-D information to 3-D in science, technology or art lessons	Worksheets without too much information or with a 'window card' to focus attention
	Red line at extreme left and use of a reading tracker
Spatial awareness: construction tasks	Use of highlighter pen to aid with scanning for main ideas
Spatial awareness: locating information on a busy worksheet	
	Provide handouts to limit copying work
Spatial awareness: visual scanning, e.g. from left to right, row by row, when reading	Keep desk as clear as possible
	Multi-sensory learning: look, copy, make it, name it, etc.
Spatial awareness: copying from the board	
	Consistent and routine approach
Shape, number, letter recognition	Verbal prompts progressing to written prompts if necessary
Motor planning: bumping into things, sequencing actions, e.g. when dressing	Provide prompts as necessary and fade them out
	Lay things out in the sequence they will be needed

ASSESSMENT AND FEEDBACK: HIGHLIGHTING STRENGTHS

As children develop, challenges may only become evident as expectations change with age. Periods of transition often highlight needs that were previously undetected, e.g. when moving from primary- to secondary-level education. Young people moving onto a GCSE programme often experience a stepwise leap in the demands on them, as they need to work more independently, monitor their own progress, plan to meet deadlines and work through a greater volume of work more quickly. Academic work usually becomes more abstract and language-based. The need to establish optimal conditions for the child's learning and being on a day-to-day basis is widely acknowledged (e.g. *Every Child Matters*, Government Green Paper, 2003).

A comprehensive psychometric assessment gives a snapshot of intellectual ability at a point in time, but the information it provides can contribute to the identification of factors that support or constrain opportunities for learning and developing.

One aim of assessment is to help the child in question discover more about their own unique style of learning. Sharing the findings and discussing them means they have an opportunity to become an observer to themselves and to take a 'meta' position on something they usually do automatically. This can mean that things they have taken for granted about themselves, e.g. 'I'm hopeless at English', can be demystified. The specific aspects of English that are difficult can be highlighted, as can the parts they are actually good at. This is used to form the basis of strategies for managing the challenges.

Teachers can be very good at identifying situations that support learning, while parents can share the positive attributes of the child that they are proud of (courage, determination, tenacity). These abilities and solutions can be incorporated into the report. Parents and children can be invited to attend a feedback session after they have received the report. They may want to invite whomever they would like to have in attendance, e.g. other family members or teachers. This meeting can also be used to discuss who the report is to be sent to. If teachers cannot attend, feedback can be shared verbally by phone with a key teacher, with permission from the family, before sending the written version. Through discussion, the child, parents and teachers can be encouraged to adapt the recommendations to suit their specific circumstances, and we emphasise the value of them discovering what they feel works in their situation and building on it. The more that children feel they have had a hand in designing their own strategies, the more ownership they will have of them and the more likelihood they will continue to evolve their own ongoing solutions. Putting the main findings of the assessment and the ideas generated for strategies into a jargon-free, child-friendly letter can also make sure the child or young person feels like an active participant in the process (Griffin and Christie, 2008).

When sharing assessment results, the child or young person can be invited to identify times when they used their talents and strengths to achieve things. These instances can be used to think with them about what that says about them as a person, and the qualities they show. These discoveries can then be moved into the future by asking how they expect they might make use of these talents in a similar way again. Thinking with them about what sorts of support they have found helpful or unhelpful in the past prepares the ground for identifying the easiest ways for them to receive support in the future.

SOME PRACTICAL INTERVENTION STRATEGIES

1. If mathematical facts are a difficulty, then allowing use of calculators or reference to multiplication tables will enable the child to practise applying their mathematical techniques with some degree of accuracy.
2. It is important not to overload them with information. A small working memory capacity will mean it is better to allow an opportunity to rehearse and store information in small chunks before adding new information.
3. If spoken information is long, such as explanations or lengthy instructions, children will grasp less of the meaning, simply because memory capacity is exceeded. Spoken information should ideally be brief, with frequent checks on understanding as well as written or other visual material to back it up.
4. Quiet environments with as few distractions as possible will be the best

learning environment. This will make sure attention is as good as it can be, and this will help with absorbing information.

5. We all do better at storing information if we think about it and evaluate it in some way first. Encouraging the child to think about thinking, e.g. by asking, 'What would help us to remember that later?' is one way of helping them to do this. Encouraging children to encode information by linking it to things they already know about that are related helps to integrate it into their existing bank of knowledge and so there are more potential 'triggers' when they are trying to recall it.

6. On a similar vein, when it seems that a child does have the information in their head but needs help locating the memory, asking questions about related topics or experience can act as a trigger for memory.

7. Underlining key words in each paragraph and linking the key words together in a funny sentence can help retrieve information from memory.

8. Children will do better at remembering information later on if they have the chance to rehearse it.

9. If giving instructions, it is helpful to ask the child to repeat what has been said in their own words, rather than simply asking if they understand. Most children are likely to say they do understand rather than put the adult to the bother of repeating themselves and rather than appearing inattentive or 'slow'.

10. Error-free learning techniques ensure that children minimise guessing at solutions to prevent discouragement and to avoid having to 'unlearn' errors. 'Errorless-learning' techniques improve recall of material by presenting a cue such as the first two letters of a word (e.g. PO_) and then presenting the full word (e.g. POTATO) prior to allowing the child to guess.

11. The vanishing-cues technique gradually decreases the cues provided in each learning trial. For example, if an individual is attempting to learn the name of a person named Diana, through pairing the name with a picture, the first presentation will pair the full name with the picture. A subsequent presentation may pair DIAN_ with the picture. The next presentation may pair DIA_ with the picture and so on. All information is initially given with less and less prompting as the teacher becomes confident that the child can get it right independently.

12. A Filofax or other diary system can be developed to suit specific needs. Different colours of notepaper can be purchased for Filofax diaries and this will provide an additional cue. When starting to use a Filofax system, it is important to have someone to discuss what is working or not working, so that it can be adapted to individual needs. Changes in circumstances may mean that changes will also be needed to the established system.

13. Mobile phones can be used to give an alarm to indicate activity changes or

to voice-record daily timetables or checklists of things needed on particular days.

14. Daily variation in memory skill is very usual. Memory skill will be affected by tiredness, mood, hunger and so on. Illness can disrupt the effectiveness of insulin regimens, affecting blood glucose levels and then potentially the ability to concentrate. Sometimes, it may be difficult to understand why a child remembers less on a particular day, but the key point is that it is unlikely to be under their direct control.

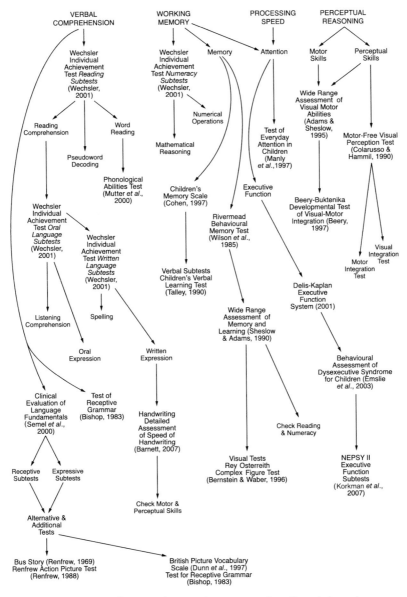

FIGURE A Different tests that can be used to assess functional domains

REFERENCES

Adams W, Sheslow D. *WRAVMA. Wide Range Assessment of Visual Motor Abilities.* Wilmington, DE: Wide Range; 1995.

Barnett A, Henderson SE, Scheib B, *et al. Developmental Assessment of Speed Handwriting.* Minneapolis, MN: Pearson; 2007.

Beery K, Buktenica A. *The Beery Developmental Test of Visual-Motor Integration.* 4th ed. Florida: Psychological Assessment Resources: 1997.

Bernstein J, Waber D. *Developmental Scoring System for the Rey-Osterrieth Complex Figure.* Lutz, FL: Psychological Assessment Resources; 1996.

Bishop D. *Test for the Reception of Grammar.* 2nd ed. Abingdon: Thomas Leach; 1983.

Cohen MJ. *Children's memory scale.* San Antonio, TX: The Psychological Corporation; 1997.

Colarusso R, Hammil D. *Motor-Free Visual Perception Test.* Revised ed. Lutz, FL: Psychological Assessment Resources; 1990.

Delis DC, Kaplan E, Kramer JH. *Delis-Kaplan Executive Function System.* San Antonio, TX: The Psychological Corporation; 2001.

Department of Health (DoH). *Every child matters.* London: The Stationery Office; 2003. Available online at: www.education.gov.uk/consultations/downloadableDocs/EveryChildMatters.pdf (accessed 18 January 2012).

Dunn L, Whetton C, Burley J. *The British Picture Vocabulary Scale.* 2nd ed. London: NFER-NELSON Publishing Company; 1997.

Emslie HC, Wilson FC, Burden V *et al. Behavioural Assessment of the Dysexecutive Syndrome in Children (BADS-C).* Bury St Edmunds: Thames Valley Test Company; 2003.

Ferguson S, Blane A, Perros P, *et al.* Cognitive ability and brain structure in type 1 diabetes: relation to microangiopathy and preceding severe hypoglycaemia. *Diabetes.* 2003; **52**(1): 149–56.

Fox M, Chen R, Holmes C. Gender differences in memory and learning in children with insulin-dependent diabetes mellitus over a 4 year follow-up interval. *J Pediatr Psychol.* 2003; **28**(8): 569–78.

Griffin A, Christie D. Taking a systemic perspective on cognitive assessments and reports. *Clin Child Psychol Psychiatry.* 2008; **13**(2): 209–20.

Holmes CS. Neuropsychological profiles in men with insulin-dependent diabetes. *Journal of Consulting and Clinical Psychology.* 1985; **54**: 386–9.

Korkman, M, Kirk, U, Kemp, S.L. *NEPSY II. Administrative Manual/Clinical and Interpretative Manual.* San Antonio, TX: Psychological Corporation; 2007.

Kovacs M, Ryan C. Verbal intellectual and verbal memory performance of youths with childhood-onset insulin-dependent diabetes mellitus. *J Pediatr Psychol.* 1994; **19**(4): 475–83.

Manly T, Robertson I; Anderson V, *et al. Test for Everyday Attention in Children.* Bury St. Edmunds: Thames Valley Test Company; 1997.

Mutter V, Hulme C, Snowling M. *Phonological Abilities Test.* London: The Psychological Corporation; 2000.

Northam E, Anderson P, Jacobs R, et al. Neuropsychological profiles of children with type 1 diabetes 6 years after disease onset. *Diabetes Care.* 2001; **24**(9): 1541–6.

Renfrew C.E. *The Action Picture Test.* 3rd ed. Oxford: C.E. Renfrew Language Test Publisher; 1988.

Renfrew C.E. *The Bus Story: a test of continuous speech.* Oxford: C.E. Renfrew Language Test Publisher; 1969.

Semel E, Wiig E, Secord W. *Clinical Evaluation Of Language Fundamentals*. 3rd UK ed. London: The Psychological Corporation; 2000.

Sheslow D, Adams W. *Wide Ranging Assessment of Memory and Learning*. Lutz, FL: Psychological Assessment Resources; 1990.

Soutor S, Rusan Chen M, Streisand R, *et al*. Memory Matters: developmental differences in predictors of diabetes care behaviours. *J Pediatr Psychol*. 2004; **29**(7): 493–505. Talley J. *Children's Auditory Verbal Learning Test*. Lutz, FL: Psychological Assessment Resources; 1990.

Wechsler, D. *Wechsler Individual Achievement Test 2nd Edition* (WIAT II). London: The Psychological Corporation; 2001.

Wilson B, Cockburn J, Baddeley A, *et al*. *The Rivermead Behavioural Memory Test* (1998). Bury St Edmunds: Thames Valley Test Company; 1985.

Regimen adherence measures

*Alan Delamater, Anna Maria Patino-Fernandez,
Elizabeth Pulgaron and Amber Daigre*

Specific measures of regimen adherence
- Self-Care Inventory (SCI) retrospective caregiver and self-report.
- Self-Care Adherence Interview (SCAI).
- Diabetes Regimen Adherence Questionnaire (DRAQ).

RETROSPECTIVE CAREGIVER AND SELF-REPORTS

Developed by La Greca *et al.* (1990), the Self-Care Inventory (SCI) is a 14-item questionnaire assessing self-perceptions of adherence to diabetes self-care recommendations over the previous 1-month period. The measure requires that respondents retrospectively rate 'how well' they have adhered to regimen recommendations (e.g. blood glucose (BG) monitoring, ketone testing, proper diet, clinic attendance, regular exercise). Responses are made on a 5-point scale, with higher scores indicating better adherence. Several researchers have reported adequate internal consistency and test-retest reliability using the SCI (Lewin, 2009; Miller and Drotar, 2003; Wysocki *et al.*, 2000). Additionally, when compared with other measures of diabetes regimen adherence (e.g. the Diabetes Self-Management Profile (DSMP), the 24-hour recall), the SCI has shown moderate to strong convergent validity as well as significant associations with glycaemic control (Greco *et al.*, 1990; Lewin, 2009).

The Self-Care Adherence Interview (SCAI) was developed by Hanson *et al.* (1987) to assess several aspects of diabetes regimen adherence (i.e. dietary behaviours, insulin adjustment, glucose testing and hypoglycaemia preparedness). The interview is administered to parents and adolescents, together or separately, and items are rated on 2- to 5-point scales. A total adherence score is calculated by adding all values, with higher scores indicating better regimen adherence. The behaviours assessed by the SCAI appear to be relatively stable, with test-retest coefficients ranging from 0.68 to 0.71 (Hanson *et al.*, 1996). Additionally, this measure shows good validity, as correlations between the SCAI and glycaemic control (i.e. HbA_{1c}) are significant and range from −0.20 to −0.28 (Hanson *et al.*, 1992).

Brownlee-Duffeck *et al.* (1987) developed the Diabetes Regimen Adherence Questionnaire (DRAQ), a retrospective self-report measure of behavioural adherence to the diabetes regimen. Respondents use a 0- to 5-point Likert scale to indicate the frequency with which they complete various self-care behaviours required for good diabetes management. Summary scores are calculated, with higher scores indicating better adherence. Good internal consistency for this measure has been reported in the range of 0.78–0.80 (Bond *et al.*, 1992; Thomas *et al.*, 1997). Research using the DRAQ has shown lower adherence scores to be correlated with negative appraisal of diabetes (Carey *et al.*, 1992) and positively correlated with better diabetes-related social problem-solving skills (Thomas *et al.*, 1997).

The DSMP was developed by Harris *et al.* (2000) as a structured interview for assessing five areas of diabetes management behaviours: (i) insulin administration and dose management; (ii) BG monitoring; (iii) exercise; (iv) diet; and (v) management of hypoglycaemia. The 23-item interview takes approximately 20–30 minutes to administer and responses are given in an open-ended manner, and are then coded by trained interviewers. All items are added to produce a total adherence score, with higher scores indicating better self-management behaviours. Investigators have reported good validity for the DSMP, with significant correlations between DSMP total scores and HbA_{1c} ($r = −0.28 − 0.60$, $p < 0.01$). Harris *et al.* (2000) reported good internal consistency of 0.76, and subsequent research has reported similarly acceptable internal consistency for child report ($\alpha = 0.72$) and parent report ($\alpha = 0.69$) (Lewin *et al.*, 2006, 2010). A recent study (Valenzuela *et al.*, 2010) provided more extensive normative data for the DSMP as well as additional information about patterns of adherence by age and gender. The DMSP has also been validated in Spanish (Valenzuela *et al.*, 2010).

TWENTY-FOUR-HOUR RECALL INTERVIEW

Johnson and colleagues developed the 24-hour recall interview approach for assessing diabetes regimen adherence (Johnson *et al.*, 1986, 1990, 1992; Reynolds *et al.*, 1990). Parents and children are interviewed separately, in person or by phone, on unscheduled occasions. The semi-structured interview covers 13 aspects of diabetes regimen adherence over the preceding 24-hour period. Generally, three interviews are conducted over 2 weeks.

Johnson *et al.* (1986, 1990, 1992) have used this methodology extensively, and results have supported its reliability and validity. Factor analysis with this method has identified four regimen factors:
1. exercise (type, duration and frequency)
2. injection (regularity, interval and timing in relation to eating)
3. diet type (carbohydrate and fat consumption)
4. frequency (eating and glucose testing).

This method uses a reference point of an ideal regimen of behaviours for children with diabetes. For example, all children's exercise is evaluated relative to a standard of three exercise periods per day; food intake is evaluated against a standard of three meals and three snacks per day, and consumption of calories based on age and gender, with 60% of calories from carbohydrate and 25% from fat; and glucose testing is evaluated relative to an ideal of four tests per day.

While this approach may limit the interpretation of adherence in individual cases, it does provide for a test of the relationship between adherence and glycaemic control across individual children. Studies have shown data obtained from the 24-hour recall interview method have significant relationships with age (older less adherent than younger), health beliefs and glycaemic control (Bond *et al.*, 1992; Johnson *et al.*, 1990, 1992; Kuttner *et al.*, 1990). Unfortunately, this method is labour-intensive in terms of both data collection and scoring, limiting its clinical utility.

ELECTRONIC METHODS

BG meters have been utilised in research as another way to gather information on regimen adherence, at least with respect to BG monitoring. Cohen *et al.* (2004) used BG meters to download the number of BG checks over the previous 10-day period (at least four blood checks per day were recommended for all children). Electronic methods have also been used to assess physical activity. For example, Faulkner *et al.* (2010) used accelerometers with a sample of adolescents to calculate the frequency of daily moderate to vigorous physical activity. Though accelerometers have been used in other paediatric populations (e.g. overweight), these investigators applied this method to paediatric diabetes, thereby allowing for more accurate reporting of exercise adherence. However, it should be noted that specific recommendations for exercise are generally not provided for children or young people with diabetes in routine clinical practice.

PHYSICIAN RATINGS

Some investigators have used ratings completed by healthcare providers to quantify regimen adherence. Jacobson *et al.* (1990) had physicians and nurses make ratings of patient adherence on a 4-point scale, ranging from poor to excellent. Acceptable reliability was obtained for ratings of adherence to diet, BG monitoring and insulin use. Psychological and family factors were found to predict regimen adherence. Anderson *et al.* (1997) modified this approach by having physicians rate adherence in the preceding 3–4 months, with respect to frequency of BG monitoring. Parental involvement in BG monitoring was significantly correlated with adherence to BG monitoring, and frequency of BG monitoring was in turn associated with gamma-hydroxybutyrate. However, the major limitation of physician rating of patient compliance is knowledge of prior adherence and glycaemic control, thereby introducing bias into such ratings. It should also be noted that health outcomes, e.g. measures of glycaemic control, may often be used as proxy measures of regimen adherence, assuming better glycaemic control implies better adherence, but this is often not the case.

REFERENCES

Anderson B, Ho J, Brackett J, *et al.* Parental involvement in diabetes management tasks: relationships to blood glucose monitoring adherence and metabolic control in young adolescents with insulin-dependent diabetes mellitus. *J Pediatr.* 1997; **130**(2): 257–65.

Bond G, Aiken L, Somerville S. The health belief model and adolescents with insulin-dependent diabetes mellitus. *Health Psychol.* 1992; **11**(3): 190–8.

Brownlee-Duffeck M, Peterson L, Simonds JF, *et al.* The role of health beliefs in the regimen adherence and metabolic control of adolescents and adults with diabetes mellitus. *J Consult Clin Psychol.* 1987; **55**(2): 139–44.

Carey M, Jorgensen RS, Weinstock RS, *et al.* Reliability and validity of the appraisal of diabetes scale. *J Behav Med.* 1992; **14**(1): 43–51.

Cohen DM, Lumley MA, Naar-King S, *et al.* Child behavior problems and family functioning as predictors of adherence and glycemic control in economically disadvantaged children with type 1 diabetes: a prospective study. *J Ped Psychol.* 2004; **29**(3): 171–84.

Faulkner M, Michaliszyn SF, Hepworth J. A personalized approach to exercise promotion in adolescents with type 1 diabetes. *Pediatr Diabetes.* 2010; **11**(3): 166–74.

Greco P, LaGreca A, Ireland S, *et al.* Assessing adherence in IDDM: a comparison of two methods [abstract]. *Diabetes.* 1990; **39**(Suppl. 1): 108A.

Hanson CL, De Guire M, Schinkel S, *et al.* Self-care behaviors in insulin-dependent diabetes: evaluative tools and their associations with glycemic control. *J Ped Psychol.* 1996; **21**(4): 467–82.

Hanson CL, De Guire M, Schinkel S, *et al.* Comparing social learning and family systems correlates of adaptation in youths with IDDM. *J Ped Psychol.* 1992; **17**(5): 555–72.

Hanson CL, Henggeler SW, Burghen GA. Model of associations between psychosocial variables and health outcome measures of adolescents with IDDM. *Diabetes care.* 1987; **10**(6): 752–8.

Harris MA, Wysocki T, Sadler M, *et al*. Validation of a structured interview for the assessment of diabetes self-management. *Diabetes Care*. 2000; **23**(9): 1301–4.

Jacobson A, Hauser ST, Lavori P, *et al*. Adherence among children and adolescents with insulin dependent diabetes mellitus over a four year longitudinal follow-up: I. The influence of patient coping and adjustment. *J Ped Psychol*. 1990; **15**(4): 511–26.

Johnson SB, Kelly M, Henretta JC, *et al*. A longitudinal analysis of adherence and health status in childhood diabetes. *J Ped Psychol*. 1992; **17**(5): 537–53.

Johnson SB, Silverstein J, Rosenbloom A, *et al*. Assessing daily management in childhood diabetes. *Health Psychol*. 1986; **5**(6): 545–64.

Johnson SB, Tomer A, Cunningham WR, *et al*. (1990). Adherence in childhood diabetes, results of a confirmatory factor analysis. *Health Psychol*. 1990; **9**(4): 493–501.

Kuttner MJ, Delamater AM, Santiago JV. Learned helplessness in diabetic youths. *J Ped Psychol*. 1990; **15**(5): 581–94.

La Greca AM, Follansbee DS, Skyler JS. Developmental and behavioral aspects of diabetes management in children and adolescents. *Children's Health Care*. 1990; **19**(19): 132–9.

Lewin AB. Validity and reliability of an adolescent and parent rating scale of type 1 diabetes adherence behaviors: the self-care inventory (SCI). *J Ped Psychol*. 2009; **34**(9): 999.

Lewin AB, Heidgerken AD, Geffken GR, *et al*. The relation between family factors and metabolic control: the role of diabetes adherence. *J Ped Psychol*. 2006; **31**(2): 174–83.

Lewin AB, Storch EA, Williams LB, *et al*. Brief report: Normative data on a structured interview for diabetes adherence in childhood. *J Ped Psychol*. 2010; **35**(2): 177–82.

Miller VA, Drotar D. Discrepancies between mother and adolescent perceptions of diabetes-related decision-making autonomy and their relationship to diabetes-related conflict and adherence to treatment. *J Ped Psychol*. 2003; **28**(4): 265–74.

Reynolds L, Johnson SB, Silverstein J. Assessing daily diabetes management by 24-hour recall interview: the validity of children's report. *J Ped Psychol*. 1990; **15**(4): 493–510.

Thomas AM, Peterson L, Goldstein D. Problem solving and diabetes regimen adherence by children and adolescents with IDDM in social pressure situations: a reflection of normal development. *J Ped Psychol*. 1997; **22**(4): 541–61.

Valenzuela J, Castro-Fernandez M, Hsin O, *et al*. Psychometric findings for a Spanish translation of the Diabetes Self-Management Profile (DSMP-Parent-Sp). *Diabetes Care*. 2010; **33**: 3–8.

Wysocki, T, Harris, M, Greco, P, *et al*. Randomized, controlled trial of behavior therapy for families of adolescents with insulin dependent diabetes mellitus. *J Ped Psychol*. 2000; **25**(1): 23–33.

Key components to consider when developing effective transition services

Janet McDonagh and Helena Gleeson

- Good therapeutic relationships among the healthcare professional, the young person and their carer is key during transition and transfer to adult services. This is, in part, achieved by the healthcare professional providing continuity of care.
- Ensuring that this therapeutic relationship is continuous into adult services requires careful consideration and should include opportunities to meet the adult team before transfer, and a member of the team or of both teams working with the young person as a transition coordinator.
- Joint clinics between paediatric and adult services do not always provide the continuity of care required and can be confusing for young people and their carers.
- Consulting with young people as a multidisciplinary team is often considered intimidating, and opportunities for one-to-one discussions are valued.
- Transition coordinator roles that span child and adult services fulfil a valuable function.
- Diabetes transition services should identify a common approach to young people with diabetes to promote continuity in diabetes management and care.
- Clinical leadership and the potential of dual or specialist qualifications and/or training in this field would assist with this.
- Psychosocial understanding is an important component of continuity in

diabetes management and care as experienced by young people and their carers.

- Ongoing involvement of carers is an important aspect of continuity in diabetes management and care at this time.
- Young people and their carers need to be provided with information as part of the preparation for transfer to adult services.
- The need for information is higher if the process of transfer to adult services is more complex.
- Joint clinics can be confusing for young people and their carers; therefore, information resources explaining their rationale and operation are indicated.
- The provision of information is an opportunity for paediatric and adult teams to work collaboratively to develop resources to support transfer.
- Structured transition programmes with individualised transition planning should be set up to support young people and their families.
- Transition planning should start in early adolescence.
- Educational programmes should address issues relating to diabetes as well as those of wider adolescence.
- Transition service should focus on becoming young person – friendly through clinic organisation and exploring different ways of communicating.
- Consultations should be organised to enable young people to be seen on their own as well as with carers.

Index